`

Food Safety Short Stories
87 Real-Life Cases

By
**Peter Overbosch, Yasmine Motarjemi
and Huub Lelieveld**

Food Safety Short Stories: 87 Real-Life Cases
By Peter Overbosch, Yasmine Motarjemi and Huub Lelieveld

This book first published 2023
Ethics International Press Ltd, UK
British Library Cataloguing in Publication Data
A catalogue record for this book is available from the British Library

Print Book ISBN: 978-1-80441-097-4
eBook ISBN: 978-1-80441-098-1

CONTENTS

Contents

Preface

The story behind the book: Food Safety Stories

It is well known that conversations in informal gatherings such as coffee breaks stimulate creativity and productivity. It was during such a meeting that we came up with the idea for this book.

It was November 2020. We were sitting at the airport in Amsterdam discussing a project on ethical practice and whistleblowing. In the course of the discussion, we recalled memories of our professional experiences. Some were foolish, others extraordinary. Each illustrated a point or gave a lesson. In this context, we thought it might be useful to collect these stories and share them in the form of a book for the younger generations or as a learning tool with trainers. Some of the stories raise also issues worth consideration for policy makers and legislators.

The idea of this book was born: a book that would capture the field experience of practitioners in their respective field, with the objective to serve as an education and training tool and that would make the training of professionals more effective. In the process, other experts joined us and generously contributed to the book with their experiences and stories.

Presented in the form of short stories, the book is a collection of unusual events or real-life situations experienced or witnessed by professionals in the food sector, with a focus on food safety, as well as related areas such as quality and legal/regulatory compliance.

The stories convey a lesson of good or bad practices in a scientific, technical, operational or management setting, or provide a lesson in ethics. They would also illustrate the kind of mishap that can happen in real life.

The objective of the stories is to provide present or future food professionals with the benefit of the work experience of other professionals. The stories also serve the lecturers/trainers in their teaching to illustrate a point and bring a lecture to life. They could also be used in classrooms for group discussions. For instance, trainers could present a story and invite participants to discuss the story and the lessons learned.

As such, the book is a complement to other existing books (e.g., Food Safety Management - a practical guide to the food industry (first edition 2014 and second edition 2022) or the Handbook of Hygiene Control in the Food Industry (2016). It is aimed at food professionals from all sectors: students, scientists, managers, trainers, professionals from the food industry or food control agencies, policy makers, certification bodies, and possibly all professionals working in the areas of risk management, public health or other sectors.

Each contribution has been anonymized to the extent possible and needed, as the objective is to support learning and focus readers' attention on the message and the points that the story would like to raise.

Yasmine Motarjemi, Peter Overbosch and Huub Lelieveld

About the authors

The idea for this book originated from discussions between three Global Harmonization Initiative members (GHI, https://www.globalharmonization.net), in the context of the GHI Working Group for Ethics in Food Safety (https://www.globalharmonization.net/wg-ethics).

Peter Overbosch worked until 2014 as Vice President of Corporate Quality Assurance, Metro Cash & Carry (based in Düsseldorf, Germany) and before that as Senior Director Quality Kraft Foods Europe, Middle East & Africa (Munich, Germany), Senior Director Quality Kraft Foods Latin America (East Hanover, NJ, USA), VP of Quality at Nabisco Inc (East Hanover, NJ, USA) and Head of Quality for Unilever Foods worldwide (Rotterdam, Netherlands). Peter is a member of the Global Harmonization Initiative (GHI), where he heads up the working group on "Ethics in Food Safety Practices", with a personal focus on establishing Food Safety Professionals as a regulated profession. Peter is a citizen of the Netherlands and holds a PhD in Chemistry from the University of Amsterdam.

Yasmine Motarjemi holds a MSc degree in Food Science and Technology from the University of Languedoc, Montpellier, France (1978) and a Doctoral degree in Food Engineering from the University of Lund, Sweden (1988). After her academic career, in 1990 she joined the World Health Organization (WHO) in Geneva as senior scientist. From 2000 to 2011, she held the position of Assistant Vice President in Nestlé and worked as the Corporate Food Safety Manager. In April 2019 she received the GUE/NGL award for Journalists, Whistleblowers and Defenders of the Right to Information, in Honour of Daphne Caruana Galizia https://www.w-t-w.org/en/award-for-journalistswhistleblowers-and-defenders-

of-the-right-to-information/   Yasmine is a member of the
Global Harmonization Initiative (GHI), and participates in the
working group on "Ethics in Food Safety Practices, leading
an initiative on legislation and practices regarding Whistle-
Blowing.

Prof. dr. h.c. **Huub Lelieveld** is President of the Global
Harmonization Initiative (GHI), Founder and Past-President
of the European Hygienic Engineering and Design Group
(EHEDG). He is also a Fellow of the International Academy of
Food Science and Technology (IAFoST). Formerly, at Unilever,
he was responsible for hygienic processing and plant design
and novel processing technologies.

Chapter One

Food safety management and whistleblowing

1.1 Letter to the CEO

It was in the days before globally recognized Food Safety (FS) certifications had become the norm in the food industry and before Hazard Analysis Critical Control Points (HACCP) was a leading FS principle in the legislation of many countries around the world. A consumer wrote to the Chief Executive Officer (CEO) of a European company operating around the world, along the following lines:

> I love this particular product of your company. Now, I am about to travel to a south-eastern Asian country for a vacation. Your product is on the market there too, I know, produced locally. As the product is potentially vulnerable to microbial contamination, I am asking you whether it is as safe there as it is here in your (and my) country?

The Public Relations (PR) department suggested that the only possible answer was a simple "yes," but the CEO felt there was more to it and gave the letter to his senior technical manager responsible for common systems within the company, with the following questions: (i) how exactly should we answer this letter? (ii) if our answer is "yes" (it is as safe there as it is here), how can we be so sure? and (iii) if our answer really is "no" or "don't know" (never mind what we actually answer to the consumer), what do we need to get to "yes."

The technical manager made inquiries in the Asian country mentioned and decided that - on an ad hoc basis - the letter could indeed be answered "yes," but he also realized that this might not necessarily be true for all the company's products in all the countries they operated in, if only because there was no way for him to be sure. Things needed to get organized, not on a market-by-market and factory-by-factory basis, with company experts assisting faraway factories as needed and on-demand, but on a much more systematic basis.

Local operating units typically jealously guarded their independence from the company's international head office and argued that de facto standards were simply different in different parts of the world and that they knew the accepted and appropriate conditions for their markets better than head office ever would. Not all things should be measured by European standards, they felt, and nobody should be under the illusion that they could get to a state of "zero risk," not even in Europe, but certainly not everywhere in the world.

While there seemed to be an element of realism there, it would also mean that the consumer's letter could never be answered with a simple "yes." It could only be a "that depends." This was felt to be unacceptable and while the "zero risk" point was well taken, the central senior technical manager told the operating units bluntly: "in this company, we will not have differential kill rates around the world" (the PR department made sure the message was not to be repeated in this form).

That started the corporate Quality Assurance/Food Safety (QA/FS) initiative, with global technical and systems standards being issued, training and audits organized, central incident management being involved whenever things went off the rails, and regular reporting to senior leadership. By the time HACCP was introduced into legislation around the world and companies needed to be certified in accordance with globally recognized standards, they were ready. All because a consumer wrote a letter (and management was smart enough to think through the implications and organize follow-up).

1.2 Employee negligence or management failure?

In 2002, as part of an internal audit, I visited an infant formula factory together with one of my colleagues. He was the lead auditor and an expert in good manufacturing practice. He was particularly skilled at identifying production problems that can pose a risk to food safety.

We entered a hall where the product was mixed in a large container, with the help of a shaft. The axle was leaning on the boarder of the vessel and scratching the bowl as it turned. During the process, due to friction, metal dust was spilling into the product. Very quickly, my colleague saw the problem and raised the issue with the factory quality manager who was following us. He replied: "Yes, you are right, during your last visit, 4 years ago, you noted the same issue!"

My colleague met with the plant manager and he immediately fired the quality manager.

Discussion and key learnings

This story raises many questions. First, we cannot only rely on audits or inspections to ensure food safety. Audits or inspections, carried out periodically, are the only measures "to verify" if preventive measures are observed, in this case, hygienic engineering and maintenance.

The only guarantee of food safety is to ensure that staff is well informed and trained, committed to product safety, and have the time and resources to do their job. If this is not the case, they should be allowed to speak up without fear of reprisals. The accountability of each level of management needs to be clarified and specified in their job descriptions.

Additionally, when there is an audit, the identified gaps, and the required corrective actions, as well as the time frame for these to be carried out, need to be documented in a report. Sometimes, as in this case, the problem may be so critical that the operation needs to be stopped and the problem corrected immediately. The plant manager should ensure with the quality manager that follow-up measures have been taken. Future audits should also verify that past identified gaps have been addressed adequately.

Also, when such events occur, before dismissing the person in charge, it is important to investigate why such a problem had lasted for several years (root cause analysis). How is it that the plant manager did not supervise and ensure that corrective measures were taken? The cause of noncompliances, be it complacencies or resource problems, needs to be reported to the top management.

Finally, inquiries should be made if the problem could occur elsewhere in the company. Were there other vessels with the same technical problem? Were equipment suppliers aware of the problem? The story does not tell, but it is advised not to fire staff before the root causes of issues are known, and accountabilities are determined.

Further reading

- Lelieveld, H., Gabric, D., Holah, J. (Eds.), 2016. Handbook of Hygiene Control in the Food Industry. Woodhead Publishing.
- Motarjemi, Y., Wallace, C., 2014. Incident management and root cause analysis Chapter 40. In: Motarjemi, Y., Lelieveld, H. (Eds.), Food Safety Management, a Practical Guide for Food Industry. Elsevier.

1.3 A question of professionalism, integrity, and courage

In the company that I worked it was taboo to say that resources and/or expertise was lacking. Anyone who would dare to say so would fall in disgrace. However, being the corporate food safety manager, I had to raise it, when necessary. Perhaps unsurprisingly, this was not well received and I suffered the consequences.

It is reported that one day, in another country, the King, escorted by his generals, visited a military hospital where my father worked. He was a surgeon colonel and the director of the hospital. The King asked my father what he needed for the hospital. He answered: "We need more qualified nurses." The King ordered the generals to follow up on this request. After the King left, the generals jumped on my father and reprimanded him for raising this issue.

Reportedly, my father replied: "If you wish, you can demote me and take away my military status; but I remain, first and foremost, a physician, and that you cannot take away from me!"

In my own situation, after multiple attempts to raise awareness about the issues surrounding food safety management in my company, I lost my job. I remembered the words of my father. I said to myself, "They took my job away from me, but they can't take away my profession and the fact that I am still a food safety and public health professional." It was then that I decided to blow the whistle on the abuses in food safety management, for the sake of public health.

Discussion and key learnings

This story is not about the King but about my father, who had the courage to speak the truth, to stand up to bullying, and to put public health above his career. It is also about the heritage that we leave to our children, that is the model that we show to future generations. It is about resilience and standing for our principles, professionalism, and dignity.

1.4 Leadership responsibility of food safety managers

I was working as the corporate food safety manager in a multinational company. One day, a new Director of Quality was appointed as my boss. His focus was on the business, even at the expense of consumers' health and safety. For instance, he was not paying attention to consumer complaints about potentially dangerous products, and he was unwilling to have raw materials monitored for possible contamination. Not only he was giving wrong advice, he was also preventing me from doing my job. Professional frustration on my side had been building up for some time, when one day, when I couldn't stand this situation any longer and I found myself at a crossroad in my life.

Should I report my boss's dysfunctional behaviour and the dire situation of the department to senior management, or keep quiet and put up with what was going on? Accepting the status quo involved the risk of a serious incident endangering the health of consumers or the reputation of the company. On the other hand, knowing the culture of the company, I knew that calling out my boss could get me dismissed.

It was a difficult decision to make, but a memory of an encounter that I had with some of our product development managers, whom I had instructed about safety aspects in product design, helped me decide.

One day, one of our operating companies reached out to my department for approval of a new product they had developed. It was an ice cream, where the wooden stick had been replaced by a glass stick, with a liquid solution that changed color. It was supposed to be attractive to children. Of course, immediately we vetoed the product. After a while the operating company came back with the same idea but had replaced the glass stick with a plastic one. After verification, we discovered the solution contained a carcinogenic substance and, on the package, a strong warning was given to consumers. Naturally, again, we strongly objected and the project was abandoned.

A few months later, I was giving a course on food safety to project managers in the ice cream business. I advocated for food safety and advised them that during product development they had to take into account all potential food safety issues and design out any potential risks. As an example of bad practice, I referred to the idea of replacing the normal wooden stick with glass and confronted them: "How could you think of producing such an ice cream? Had you lost your mind?" Then, one of the participants raised his hand. He said that this product had been designed in his market and that many opposed its production, but that they had been fired. Later, I learned that he himself was ostracized for opposing the design of the product. I replied: "Whatever happens to you, you must never accept products that you know are dangerous to consumers."

So, when I had to decide what to do, I remembered this event and realized that the problem was a pervasive "business over safety" culture. It was not just me having my own frustrations. Now could I, the person responsible for food safety, stay in my position and maintain credibility without openly opposing and reporting such situations? So, I made my report and suffered the consequences I feared. Nevertheless, to this day, I do not regret my decision.

Discussion and key learnings

Being in charge of food safety in a company, small or large, you will be confronted with situations that require you to stand your ground, in some cases against formidable internal opposition. If food safety is not a real core value within the company culture at such moments, your credibility, your authority, and indeed your continued employment may be at stake. Blowing the whistle at such moments may be unavoidable from a perspective of personal responsibility and integrity, but it may also have very negative personal consequences.

Because the importance of food safety and the critical role of food safety managers in a potentially very challenging environment is increasingly recognized, the regulatory framework around the protection of whistleblowers is slowly changing, and more and more countries are legislating for their protection.

Further reading

- Motarjemi, Y., June 1, 2014a. Whistleblowing: Food Safety and Fraud. Food Safety Magazine. https://www.food-safety.com/ articles/3670-whistleblowing-food-safety-and-fraud.
- Motarjemi, Y., 2014b. Human factors in food safety management. In: Motarjemi, Y., Lelieveld, H. (Eds.), Food Safety Management: A Practical Guide for the Food Industry. Academic Press, Waltham, MA.
- Motarjemi, Y., 2023. Whistleblowing: an essential element of public health and food safety management. In: Andersen, V., Lelieveld, H., Motarjemi, Y. (Eds.), Food Safety Management. A Practical Guide for the Food Industry, second ed. Academic Press. Waltham MA.

1.5 QA/FS and senior management; good intentions may go wrong

In my working life, I have had the privilege of working with a number of very experienced senior managers in large food companies. Most of them, typically coming from financial or marketing backgrounds, were supportive of QA/FS programs but not familiar with what we were actually doing. They also felt that food safety should not be used as a competitive advantage "we are not going to tell the general public that our product is safer than our competitor's, even when that might be true" and that the focus of the company should be on those activities that drive the business. Asked why quality and safety had not been mentioned at all in a long-term visionary plan for our company, one CEO told me that "quality is a given" and he did not seem to appreciate my question as to who had given it to him.

Another CEO in another company informed me that he wanted "no more public recalls," after we indeed had a few of them in the recent past. My answer that we were working on it and that I was confident that over time we would significantly reduce the risk if we continued to implement our programs was not well received. "You did not understand me," he said, "I want no more public recalls." With the help of some other senior managers, he was brought to see reason and afterward continued to be supportive of our efforts. One of his lieutenants later told me that he had explained QA to his boss "it's like an insurance policy," he said, "QA doesn't drive the business, but we need to spend the money, to keep safe." I did tell him that we are the exact opposite; insurance allows you to continue doing what you are doing, but it will pay out when things go wrong. QA tells you that you must change your ways, and we don't pay out when things go wrong after all.

A very proactive CEO at yet another company announced that he would introduce a gamechanger, a measure that would show everybody the company's commitment to quality and safety and make it count to his staff and their reports. The end-of-year bonuses would be linked to recalls - if one occurred in your area, that would impact negatively on your bonus. The idea was that we would all focus more on good practices and prevention, but that was not exactly what happened.

The Senior Vice President (SVP) of Operations that I worked with at the time informed me that from now there would be no more recalls issued, unless agreed with one of his product-sector VPs. There seemed to be not much point in escalating this discussion at that moment and things seemed to work for a while (obviously we did not have that many recalls), until one day I was informed that we had a serious problem. One of our products contained an allergen, which in that particular batch was not declared on the label. Consumers had complained of relatively serious allergic reactions and some had informed the authorities.

The situation could not be clearer; a product was mislabeled, therefore illegal; there were serious complaints, and the authorities could be on our doorstep at any moment. This was a textbook public recall. Before instructing the country organization to initiate the recall, I dutifully tried to reach the sector VP, but no luck. And so, the recall was initiated, the general public and authorities informed, emergency messages sent to the sector VP and to his boss, the SVP of Operations. He was furious. Asked why his VP was not contactable at the time and what he felt should have been done differently under these circumstances, he eventually calmed down and we were able to refocus his attention to preventive QA/FS measures instead of prevention of recalls per se. The recall-related bonus measure silently disappeared a bit later.

Discussion and key learnings

The relationship between QA/FS managers and top management is not always easy. The people involved typically come from very different backgrounds; QA/FS does not drive business, cannot be used as a marketing tool, and does not speak in financial terms. Still, it is essential that senior management, who typically are from marketing/finance backgrounds, but not well versed in, e.g., microbiology or HACCP, understands enough about QA/FS to make the kind of decisions that only they can. For QA/FS in large companies, it is therefore essential that they have board-level representation, separate from, e.g., operations or marketing, to avoid important potential conflicts of interest being decided, and potentially hidden from view, below board level.

In this story, the recall-bonus link is a clear example of good intentions with unexpected negative consequences, a perverse incentive to try and avoid even clear case recalls. The intention was to focus people's attention on preventive measures, but that was not sufficiently explained, and it came without additional supportive measures (e.g., "we will invest in a company-wide certification effort," or "we will review all our HACCP plans again the coming two years, with the help of external experts").

There have been cases, however, where a link between recalls and bonuses was introduced with no intention at all to emphasize preventive measures, just suppressing the number of recalls. In some cases, that then led to, e.g., a reduction in the programs to monitor contaminants in raw materials.

The conclusion at this point is that linking bonuses to recalls introduces counter- productive incentives into a company's food safety practices. Managers need to be encouraged to do the right things and only be (financially) sanctioned if they are found to have violated company rules or principles or neglected their duties.

1.6 What lessons from the Great Wall of China?

When I joined the World Health Organization in 1990, one of the first subjects I was asked to work on was health education in food safety. At that time, a lot of work had already been done in the department and several publications on the subject were in preparation.

The central point of these publications was that biological or chemical sciences and technology, i.e., technical data, are not sufficient to manage product safety. Equal attention needs to be paid to human factors, i.e., education and/or training of operators, whether managers, workers, food handlers, or caregivers, and these need to be based on social and anthropological information.

The idea was that in order to convince and motivate operators of any category to follow recommended safety measures or do their work in a flawless manner, it is necessary to understand their perceptions, constraints, living, and working conditions and also ensure that the recommended measures or instructions are feasible and culturally acceptable.

Later, working in food industry, but also studying incidents in other risk sectors such as aviation, I gained first-hand experience and a deeper insight into the importance of the human factor in food safety management. I realized how much compliance of staff depends on company culture, working conditions, attitude and ethics of the employees themselves, and the behavior of managers.

Recently, I read a story in National Geographic that reminded me of this aspect of food safety management and illustrates the importance of human factors in risk management.

For centuries, nomadic herders living in the steppe territories bordering northern China have posed a threat to the Chinese population.

As a defense strategy, at various times, but especially in the 16th and 17th centuries, during the Ming Dynasty, a wall about 21,000 km long was built. It is known as the "Great Wall of China." The Chinese rulers were convinced that the wall would protect their people from the aggression of nomads, including the Mongols. However, despite this impressive military construction, the Great Wall did not fully achieve its main purpose.

It is explained that the men who guarded the wall lived in extremely difficult conditions. They lacked food and warm clothing and suffered from hunger, cold, and wind. They were separated from their families for months or even years - a situation that undermined their morale and created mistrust. The guard troops were not dedicated to their task.

There are several accounts of how the guards did not perform their duties or failed to alarm when the Mongols attacked. Some even fled without resistance. Sometimes they had friendly contacts with the enemies or traded with them. Sometimes they even colluded with them.
These conditions meant that, despite the ingenious military structure, nomads could scale the wall with hooks and enter Chinese territory without much defense from the guards.

Discussion and key learnings

Historical events provide valuable life lessons. Great walls and military tactics will all be to no avail without the human factor. The lesson for food safety management is the same:

All the technology and science will not guarantee product safety if the operators are not motivated, do not have a sense of ethics and professionalism, or if they have to work under threat and duress. The recent focus on "food safety culture" seems to formally recognize the towering importance of the human factor in the success of food safety systems. That is great progress, but these lessons really go back to ancient times.

Further reading

- Motarjemi, Y., 2014. Human factors in food safety management. In: Motarjemi, Y., Lelieved, H. (Eds.), Chapter 37 in Food Safety Management. A Practical Guide for the Food Industry, pp. 975-986.
- The Great Wall of China's long legacy, National Geography. https://www.nationalgeographic.com/history/history-magazine/article/the-great-wall-of-china.
- WHO, 2000. Foodborne Disease : A Focus for Health Education. World Health Organization, 9241561963. https://apps.who.int/iris/handle/10665/42428.

1.7 Get your HACCP certificate, hurry, hurry!

Some years ago, I worked as a quality and HACCP systems auditor. During the audits, I used to observe the reactions of people when asking how they manage the HACCP system. I often found they had interesting views, but most of all they wished the auditor to see as little as possible and to discover as few noncompliances as possible.

In one case, I was auditing a HACCP system at an operating unit of a large food company and I asked the person in charge to present their hazard analysis. It got complicated from the very start, since the site had neither identified and assessed all relevant risks nor their causes or, as a result, defined necessary preventive measures. Furthermore, the HACCP documentation was not systematized and did not provide traceability for certain record sheets and work instructions.

Actual practice was much better, but people responsible for individual processes had difficulty explaining their procedures, since the way they worked was inconsistent with the actual documentation. Still, they tried all sorts of arguments to convince me that their systems and practices were compliant with HACCP principles/systems.

When I reported my findings including inconsistencies with the HACCP system, factory management showed indignation and refused to accept it. They tried to convince me they were in the process of harmonizing HACCP documentation and asked for my understanding. However, my findings stood and as an auditor, I simply had to follow the official standards. This production site failed the audit.

Shortly afterward, the European inspectors also discovered quite a number of inconsistencies. At a follow-up audit later,

I found the situation to be much better and the awareness around HACCP system to be at a much higher level.

Discussion and key learnings

The parent company had marked this production site as a source for export to foreign markets, so they needed to get their certificates ASAP and prepared the necessary HACCP documentation hastily and apparently without any substantial support from the parent company. That is not always the case, many larger food companies issue standard HACCP and general QA system templates for their subsidiaries for them to adapt to local conditions and implement. Not here.

In this case, those responsible for the overall HACCP system and individual processes were aware of the weaknesses in documentation, which was not fully consistent with practice, but they did not want to admit it.

The main issue is that, in general, documentation is often perceived as an administrative paperwork and not as a means of communication among HACCP team members or as a basis for review and reflection. Documentation is also important in case of investigation of an adverse event, or inspection, certification to prove that what is necessary has been carefully considered and implemented. It is also important in case of a change in the process or ingredients and evaluation of possible modifications to be brought.

Additionally:

- Multinational companies that do not provide their operating units with standard HACCP and QA system templates are missing a huge opportunity and opening the door to inconsistent practices.

- Under pressure (to start production for export and get their certificates), people will cut corners and try to defend clearly inconsistent and noncompliant systems to auditors.
- Auditors need to remain calm and focused under pressure. The auditee may not always be happy, but the integrity of the audit and the credibility of a certificate come first. A negative audit or inspection evaluation may in the short term upset but in the long term it may serve the company and protect consumers.
- The importance of documentation needs to be clearly understood (and therefore often better explained) to the management of businesses.

1.8 Food safety: a corporate social responsibility

The company for which I was working was importing honey from an Asian country and was using it in various products, such as infant cereal. In the early 2000s, we learned that the imported honey in Europe contained a prohibited antibiotic, chloramphenicol, and this was used in several of our products in Europe.

At the time, I was working in the mother company as the Corporate Food Safety Manager. The crisis management team was immediately convened, the situation was reviewed, and instructions for the management of the crisis were prepared. Our scientists provided instructions for in-house analysis of the products. We required recall of products that were in violation of the legislation. In one of the European markets, these instructions met fierce opposition on the part of a country Quality Manager. An eventual recall would cause his operating company considerable financial loss, and he had to face the reprimand of his higher-level management for the incident. He objected to the instructions. Among other things, he viewed that the method of analysis was too sensitive and likely to detect the presence of chloramphenicol at low levels, where authorities would not detect it with their less sensitive method.

As a follow-up to this crisis, we decided to conduct a worldwide survey of chloramphenicol in our products to ensure that worldwide all products are compliant and to investigate if such a violation occurs elsewhere. We detected the use of chloramphenicol in some Asian and Latin American countries, in particular in milk products. Hence, we recommended the testing of the raw materials and rejecting noncompliant milk and re-examining the practice of suppliers.

Sometime after, I was attending a sumptuous conference banquet. I sat at the table of some Technical Directors. I was happy with our crisis management and our proactive actions to clean up our products from possible contamination. It was then that one of the technical directors working in Latin America said angrily: I am very cross with you!

I asked: Why? This is not the way to manage antibiotics in milk and dairy products! So how should we have managed it, in your opinion? You should dilute the contaminated milk with noncontaminated milk! he said. Certainly, in this way, you may reduce the level of contamination to perhaps an undetectable level. However, what about the supplier who would continue with this practice and sell to other companies? And what about the fact that consumers may be exposed to this milk, viewed as inappropriate by public health authorities? What about our corporate social responsibility and ensuring that the raw material on the market is free from contamination? What about if one of the contaminated batches escapes our dilution efforts and we are caught with such a violation?

A few years later my company audited a supplier of peanut butter. It was found that the peanut butter was produced in unsanitary conditions. We silently changed suppliers but let the offending supplier continue with his unsanitary practices. As a consequence, a major outbreak of salmonellosis happened in North America, sickening some 700 people. Nine persons died. My company proudly announced that it had audited the company and not used its peanut butter.

Discussion and key learnings

Regulatory standards are established for the protection of public health or consumer rights and need to be respected by companies. Ad hoc or short-term exposure to certain prohibited agents at trace levels may not necessarily pose a significant health risk to consumers and it may be unnecessary to recall affected products for safety reasons. However, allowing such practices to continue will contribute to an overall unacceptable exposure of consumers. Therefore, noncompliant suppliers need to be identified and corrected.

The decision about what is acceptable or not should be taken by regulatory authorities as they are in the position to consider the overall exposure of consumers and long-term implications.

Regarding the use of prohibited chemicals, it is not the amount of contaminant present, which is per se a violation, but its use. Hence, using a sensitive method of analysis is important for detecting suppliers who violate the law and may in the future pose a serious problem.

Following a crisis, it is important to follow up to verify that the contaminants or malpractice is not occurring elsewhere in raw material, products, or other markets.

A question that remains open is what is the social responsibility of a company that finds critical food safety issues with a supplier. Up to now, companies typically walk away from such suppliers, discontinuing their business with them, but implicitly allowing the dangers to public health to continue. Taking a public stand in those cases invites the risk of litigation, especially if the company that blows the whistle on a supplier is from another country - the supplier may enjoy a "home advantage." Also, suppliers may object to audits if they do not want to see the results ending up in the public domain. In such cases, it is easier for both parties to say nothing and go their separate ways - at the expense of food safety and public health.

Further reading

- Motarjemi, Y., 2014. Crisis management. In: Motarjemi, Y., Lelieveld, H. (Eds.), Food Safety Management; a Practical Guide for the Food Industry. Academic Press, Waltham, pp. 1037-1063.
- Tenud, R., Brück, W.M., Motarjemi, Y., Forthcoming. Management of chemical contaminants. In: Andersen, V., Lelieveld, H., Motarjemi, Y. (Eds.), Food Safety Management. A Practical Guide for the Food Industry, second ed. Academic Press.

1.9 The hermit and the whistleblower

Sometimes we find ourselves in a difficult situation and wonder what to do; whatever the decision, it can backfire. We are damned. The decision-making process becomes an ordeal.

A few years ago, when I was responsible for food safety in a large food company, I found myself in such a situation. I witnessed food safety management practices that appeared unacceptable to me. I could foresee the risk of an imminent incident and possible harm to consumers. Yet, I found myself to be powerless to change the situation. No matter what I said, my superior, the Quality Management Director, would not listen and discouraged me from raising the subject again.

The only thing I felt I could do was to complain to the top management. However, strangely enough, despite the company's policy, i.e., its code of conduct, which encourages staff to report any problems, Human Resource (HR) asked me to withdraw my complaint. "Here the boss is always right!", the HR Director said. This was not the first time I had received a warning. I remember that a few months after I joined the company and protested against what I saw as misconduct and bad practices, the secretary of our department gave me the sculpture of the three wise monkeys, meaning "see no evil, hear no evil, speak no evil."

So, the question for me was what to do? I considered two options: One was to insist on reporting the issues, knowing that I would run the risk of being sanctioned. The other option was to follow HR's advice, withdraw my complaint, play the three wise monkeys, and go with the flow.

It was a difficult decision to make. In one case, I feared losing my job when I could not afford it, or having my life made miserable; in the other, I had to compromise my professional integrity and live with the shame of failing my responsibilities to consumers. I was agonizing over this decision when I recalled a childhood memory. Then, the decision became clear.

I was about 6 or 7 years old. From time to time, my parents would take me on a picnic to the mountains. Near the picnic site, there was a place called "father of the mountain." For a long time, an old man had been living there, alone and simply, in a hut made of wood and mud. We, the children, found him weird and mysterious. We liked to play around his place and, from time to time, to tease him.

At that critical moment in my career, I saw his face before me: white hair, pale, wrinkled skin, unshaven. He had tattered clothes and looked poor, living on almost nothing. Nevertheless, he seemed composed, serene, and at peace with himself and the world. I looked at my own situation: I was relatively well off: a good salary, good living conditions, a luxurious car, living in a beautiful and prosperous country, and yet I felt miserable. No doubt, better to be poor and happy than rich and miserable.

This is how my life as a whistleblower started. I resubmitted my complaint and endured the expected consequences. But I never regretted my decision.

Discussion and key learnings

In a well-run company with a positive food safety culture, the need for whistleblowing rarely arises. Managers comply with responsible company/organizational policies and are committed to food safety. Employees who observe a threat to food safety, whether deliberate or accidental, are encouraged and enabled to report it safely without fearing retaliation and they are heard.

In contrast, when food safety personnel, or any other employee for that matter, report critical issues, and subsequently they are sanctioned, harassed, or dismissed because of that, we may speak of a negative food safety culture. When employees are silenced by fear of reprisals, food safety problems may go unnoticed and remain unaddressed. Employees working under duress may also be unable to fulfil their responsibilities. Therefore, I would argue, such situations should be considered as critical violations of food safety.

However, the importance of whistleblowing in the food sector has not yet received the same degree of recognition as in the financial sector, where many countries have enacted specific laws for the promotion of whistleblowing and protection of whistleblowers. Even in these cases, employees are still reluctant to speak out because they risk their jobs and careers or face severe retaliation and have difficulty obtaining redress.

Further reading

- Griffith, C., Motarjemi, Y., 2023. Human factor. In: Andersen, V., Lelieveld, H., Motarjemi, Y. (Eds.), Food Safety Management. A Practical Guide for the Food Industry, second ed. Academic Press, Waltham MA.
- Motarjemi, Y., 2023. Whistleblowing: an essential element of public health and food safety management. In: Andersen, V., Lelieveld, H., Motarjemi, Y. (Eds.), Food Safety Management. A Practical Guide for the Food Industry, second ed. Academic Press. Waltham MA.
- Motarjemi, Y., forthcoming. Acquiescence versus dissent in the corporate world. In: Grasso, C. (Ed.), Whistleblowers: Voices of Justice, Springer International.

1.10 Can food safety be translated into financial value?

A few years ago, in the summer, I got a call in the morning from a food business operator - the owner of a seafood restaurant I occasionally consulted for. When he came into the restaurant kitchen in the morning, he found that one of his refrigerators had stopped working during the night. The control thermometer was showing 22°C. Considering the contents of the fridge (fish and other seafood), I advised him to discard the affected goods as a precautionary measure to prevent any health risks for his restaurant's guests.

He was shocked and upset, considering the economic value of the goods in the refrigerator. So, I put the situation in different perspective and explained to him that if he rejects the food in the fridge, that will be the only cost. If he doesn't, maybe nothing will happen, but if he takes a risk and uses those goods as ingredients in his dishes and then his guests contract a foodborne illness at his restaurant, he will be responsible and be fined, and/or even shut down temporarily, by food safety authorites. This will be a stain on the reputation of his restaurant and he will lose a lot of guests and revenue. However, his fixed costs including the high monthly rent (which was double the cost of the fridge contents) will continue.

I made a rough calculation of the potential damages in case of foodborne illness and left the final decision to him. In the end, he decided not to sell the fish and other seafood from the broken fridge, but also not to reject and destroy it. Instead, he had a fish picnic for his relatives. I was not informed of this until after the picnic because he wanted me to know I was wrong. Fortunately, there was no outbreak of foodborne illness.

Discussion and key learnings

While working (professionally and academically) with food handlers and food business operators, I have found that the majority of them are much more "money sensitive" than "health sensitive." That is, when discussing food safety issues with others, it is important to understand what drives the person we are dealing with and to adapt the language of communication to their values. In the case briefly described earlier, we can see that the health and safety issues were not "real" to him, but the money aspect was.

However, explaining things in the (financial) terms that he understood did not turn him into a health-sensitive food business owner/ handler. Even though I prevented the food safety risk to the restaurant guest, I could not foresee him having a fish picnic in his private circle because he did not ask me. And because (thankfully) nothing happened, he was even more convinced that my advice was exaggerated and he could have sold the goods from the broken fridge without any negative consequences.

1.11 "Off with their heads!"

On an assignment in the Pacific Island to train food inspectors, one of the weekends, we went on a semi-professional trip to explore how the bush people lived and prepared food. During a meal we had with a family, the hosts told us about a custom of their ancestors. They told us that - in the old times - when houses were built, it was customary to put a human head under the main pillar of the house - a sacrifice to appease the powers that otherwise might harm the new dwelling. For this purpose, a specific family was designated. Each time a house was built, a member of this family lost their head.

The islanders had discontinued the practice long ago, but the way some companies use their QA/FS function seems to bear some odd similarities in this respect, and I witnessed such a situation in action.

The company of which I am speaking - and where I worked for 10 years - proudly proclaimed that: "Food safety is not negotiable! Food safety is a priority! Food safety is everyone's responsibility! The quality of food depends on the quality of management!"

However, food safety managers had little authority in relevant decision-making processes, and risk assessment and prevention, in the course of proactive food safety management, was simply not on the cards.

Purchasing looked for the cheapest raw material on the international market without considering safety issues, or how we could audit remote suppliers. They thought that testing some samples was a reliable way of controlling food safety and could not be persuaded otherwise. Similarly, decisions were made about purchasing and managing factories, without considering the state of these facilities and the time and investments needed to improve infrastructure and food safety management. Contract manufacturers were sometimes chosen without considering their competence in food safety management. The same was true for the marketing of products. In one case, preparation instructions were changed, and storage of the prepared product was extended for marketing reasons, which led to a fatal incident.

In short, business decisions were routinely made without considering food safety implications.

So, what were QA/FS managers for in this company? They had responsibilities but no authority. They often had no job description, so people had to guess what exactly they could/not do and they were not happy.

Management was often reluctant to take preventive measures, such as screening raw materials, auditing suppliers, or even recalling contaminated/defective products, if they believed that the contamination would not be detected. They preferred to take risks and then expected the QA/FS department to bail them out when things went wrong, as if the QA/FS staff had a magic wand that they could wave to turn a poor- quality food into a safe, high-quality product. If QA/FS could not, they would be held responsible for the debacle and be blamed.

One of my colleagues wanted to leave this QA/FS environment and expressed his frustration with the way product quality was handled: GIGA (garbage in, garbage out).

So, in the years I worked at this company, I had the impression that the QA/FS staff were like those poor islanders, they were there to appease the outside world : "we have this wonderful QA/FS organization and they keep our products safe", but had no real authority in keeping things safe. If something happened, their role was to have their heads "cut off."

Discussion and key learnings

- The QA/FS function's responsibility is (should be) to assess and manage risks on behalf of the company. They need to be involved in product development, raw material procurement, hygienic design of equipment and facilities, testing protocols, etc., at an early stage to be effective. General management needs to recognize that and create an environment where QA/FS is allowed, encouraged, and supported to do their job.
- QA/FS need a clear and agreed job description (like everybody else); it is an essential part of an environment where QA/FS is allowed, encouraged, and supported to do their job.
- Testing final product to assure safety is unreliable and old-fashioned. The development of HACCP started with a recognition of that simple fact.
- Sh*t will happen but when things go wrong, it is not necessarily QA/FS's fault. Taking the blame is not uniquely in their job description. It is essentially in everybody's.
- Company executives need to be trained to have an awareness of food safety management commensurate to their responsibilities. They need to understand not only the principles but also the limits of their knowledge. Furthermore, they need to understand the potential consequences of decisions that only they can make.

Further reading

- Griffith, C.J., Livesey, K.M., Clayton, D.A., 2010. Food safety culture: the evolution of an emerging risk factor? British Food J. 112 (4), 426e438.

- Motarjemi, Y., 2014a. Whistleblowing: Food Safety and Fraud. Food Safety Magazine. Available at: https://www.food-safety. com/articles/3670-whistleblowing-food-safety-and-fraud.
- Motarjemi, Y., 2014b. Human factors in food safety management: a practical guide for the food industry, Chapter 37. In: Motarjemi, Y., Lelieveld, H. (Eds.), Food Safety Management. Academic Press, Waltham, MA, pp. 975-986.
- Motarjemi, Y., 2023. Whistleblowing: an essential element of public health and food safety management. In: Andersen, V., Lelieveld, H., Motarjemi, Y. (Eds.), Food Safety Management. A Practical Guide for the Food Industry, second ed. Academic Press. Waltham MA.

Chapter Two

Communication, education and (mis)information

2.1 Moving a mountain: changing perceptions on childhood diarrhoea

In 2011, in a famous scientific journal, an article was published on child mortality (Moore et al., 2011). The article discussed the causes of diarrhoea in small children without mentioning the role of food contamination at all. The article frustrated me. For years, I and other food safety professionals have been raising awareness about the role of food contamination in childhood diarrhoea and trying to correct this omission in global policies (Motarjemi et al., 1993).

So, I wrote to the first author and asked him if he did not believe that food contamination played a role in childhood diarrhoea. The author admitted that he had made a mistake in omitting the role of food, but he justified his error by saying that he was following the policy of an international public health organization.

This event reminded me of a memory when I was on assignment in a developing country. During a roundtable discussion on the topic of childhood diarrhoea, breast-feeding and the provision of safe water were mentioned as means of prevention. However, there was no mention of educating caregivers about food hygiene. When I raised the issue of food contamination and suggested that food hygiene should also be promoted, I was met with fierce opposition. I asked what harm there would be in adding the role of food and food safety education to the actions they were taking. The answer was that this would dilute their efforts on the other measures. Only one person, out of the 10-12 people present, took my side and defended my position. He then turned to me and said: "Ma'am, I wish you lots of energy because you will have to move a mountain".

Going back to the erroneous article, the author of the article did not offer to retract his article or correct it. I shared the situation with some other public health professional colleagues. They offered to publish another article highlighting the need for an integrated approach to addressing the risk factors for childhood diarrhoea (Motarjemi et al., 2012). We did so, but unfortunately the article painting a seriously incomplete, and thereby misleading, picture of the childhood diarrhoea problem is still available and continues to mislead other scientists.

Discussion and key learnings

The role of food and food safety has been neglected for years in childhood diarrhoea prevention policies, with consequences that can be imagined. The scientific integrity and ethics of scientists are fundamental to effectively addressing public health issues and protecting the world's population. Scientists should write not only the truth, but the whole truth. Unfortunately, they sometimes prefer to take the easy path and follow the prevailing thinking, even if they know there is more to the problem at hand.

The fact that an article is published in a reputable, peer-reviewed, journal does not guarantee that it presents a balanced perspective. Peer review is not necessarily a catch-all.

Once the author freely admitted that food safety should have been included in his article, the appropriate thing to do would have been to retract/correct the article, if only for the sake of the ongoing struggle against childhood diarrhoea. It would have helped in building policies and programs in many countries. As things stand, the original article continues to be a reference on the subject, supporting deep-rooted misperceptions that are difficult to eradicate.

References

- Moore, S., Lima, A., Guerrant, R., 2011. Preventing 5 million child deaths from diarrhoea in the next 5 years. Nat. Rev. Gastroenterol. Hepatol. 8, 363-364.
- Motarjemi, Y., Kaferstein, F.K., Moy, G.G., Quevedo, F., 1993. Contaminated weaning food: a major risk factor for diarrhoea and associated malnutrition. Bullet. World Health Organ. 71 (1), 79-92.
- Motarjemi, Y., Steffen, R., Binder, H.J., September, 2012. Preventive strategy against infectious diarrhoea; a holistic approach. Gastroenterology 143 (3), 516-519.

2.2 The risks of risk communication in food safety

On the occasion of World Food Safety Day on June 7, 2021, the European Food Safety Agency launched its new risk communication campaign entitled "Choose Safe Food" to encourage people to think critically about their everyday food habits. This brought to mind my experience at the World Health Organization (WHO) in regard to fashioning a global food safety message, which presented several challenges that are discussed below.

When I joined the WHO Food Safety Unit in 1991, the Ten Golden Rules for Safe Food Preparation had already been devised by the head of the unit. The detailed rules included all of the common factors known to impact on food safety. Subsequently, WHO issued a "poster" which listed the detailed rules with no graphics. On the back of the "poster" was a message intended for national authorities to advise them to adapt the rules to the language and conditions of the country. While the poster was translated into the six official languages of WHO, few authorities appeared to adapt the rules to the culture and conditions of their country. One notable example was when a breakfast cereal company in Pakistan reproduced the Ten Golden Rules, which completely filled the back of the product box and notable in English. One might have asked, "Who was the audience?" And this is really the critical question in risk communication about food safety as so many actors are involved from production to consumption.

While widely disseminated, the Ten Golden Rules were probably not the best risk communication vehicle because most people have difficulty remembering 10 specific items. However, this basic problem was not addressed until food safety had gained some national attention. In WHO, this resulted in the establishment of the Department of Food Safety and Zoonoses. In recognizing the shortcomings of the golden rules, the WHO food safety team set out to devise a better approach for communicating basic messages on food safety.

It was agreed that the list be limited to a small number of key behaviors that people could remember and, hopefully, put into practice. They would include short explanations as to why they were important, followed by some specific examples. Relying on the advice of experts in risk communication, the WHO team debated the most important food safety behaviors and finally came to agreement. The five simple messages were launched in 2001 by WHO as the Five Keys to Safer Food, which can be summarized as:

- Keep clean
- Separate raw and cooked
- Cook thoroughly
- Keep food at safe temperatures
- Use safe water and raw materials.

This was presented in a poster that showed the five behaviors as keys and each key had a little statement about "why" and then followed by a few examples. Although the public only sees the final product, the process of formulating the Five Keys was fraught with scientific uncertainty and differences of opinion. This is illustrated in the following two examples. The first relates to a technical issue that started as a scientific matter but also raised a policy question.

Interpreting science: By the turn of the century, Hazard Analysis Critical Control Point (HACCP) was widely accepted as the best method for assuring the safety of food, but it presented a number of technical challenges. This was addressed with "Cook thoroughly" and concerned the specific advice about the temperature needed to destroy foodborne pathogens. While not mentioned in the key behavior, 70oC is stated in the "why" as the temperature that destroys foodborne pathogens. Although it is most commonly used, in actual scientific experiments, usually challenge studies, a variety of temperatures were used. However, 70oC was chosen, in part, for simplicity. But the basic question is still "Who is the audience?" Commercial operators and consumers in industrialized countries would have thermometers to measure temperature, but this advice is not universal. This also is an issue with "Keep food at safe temperatures" where the science is more uncertain. This example reveals the challenges of turning science into universal messages.

Who is the audience? The second example more directly deals with the question "Who is the audience?" As mentioned, this story was prompted by the "Chooses Safe Food" campaign. It called to mind the discussions the WHO team had related to the last of the Five Keys to Safer Food, namely "Use safe water and raw materials." This is different from the other key behaviors in that it specifies safe water. However, it was felt at the time that this was too important for public health to leave out, as diarrheal diseases related to contaminated food and water are among the leading causes of morbidity and mortality in developing countries. However, the latest WHO data suggest that this message is not as universal as one might expect, as a majority of the world's population (over 70%) now have access to safe drinking water. Consequently, this key behavior was aimed at the 30% of the world populations without safe water. In retrospect, it might have been better to simply name this key behavior "Choose safe food." For countries where safe water is a problem, one of the examples should have been "Use safe water." A more universal example would be "Wash raw fruits and vegetables", which is a critical control point in many HACCP systems. "Choose safe food" is also logically the first key behavior, as purchasing food is the first step in food preparation. From a risk communication viewpoint, "Choose safe food" encourages everyone to think about safe food, so it is perhaps the key of the key behaviors.

Discussion and key learnings

In fashioning any risk communication message in food safety, the first question that must be answered is "Who is the audience?" This includes consideration of the social, cultural, and environmental context as well as the specific goals of the communication. Is the audience interested in being educated in food safety or does the audience need only basic training in food safety?

As a global message, the Five Keys to Safer Food must be seen as an excellent universal format for risk communication in food safety. However, it is clear that it needs to be adapted at the national level before any food safety communication campaign is launched. However, the fact that the Five Keys have been translated into 88 languages, mostly without any changes, is a sign that the communication about adapting them has not been received.

Ideally, food safety managers should establish priorities for risk communication based on likely causes of foodborne disease revealed by thorough investigation of outbreaks and studies of possible risk factors.

References

- EFSA, 2021. EFSA launches "EU Choose Safe Food" campaign on World Food Safety Day, 7 June 2021. Available at: https://www.efsa.europa.eu/en/news/efsa-launches-eu-choose-safe-food- campaign-world-food-safety-day.
- Kaferstein, F., 1988. The pleasures and pitfalls of eating, World Health Magazine. Available at: https://apps.who.int/iris/bitstream/handle/10665/53104/WH-1988-Nov-p6-8-eng.pdf.
- WHO, 2001. Five Keys to Safer Food poster (88 languages). Available at: https://apps.who.int/iris/ handle/10665/66735.

2.3 Bread in times of pandemic: the fabrication of disinformation

Making informed food choices depends on having access to correct and transparent information. There is common legislation for the enforcement of consumer protection laws (ICPEN, 2021) and there are governmental bodies and consumer organizations to prevent food fraud and unethical practices in the market place. But sometimes, that is not enough.

These days, practically all communication channels, from television to social networks, are overflowing with coronavirus information, sometimes solid, but sometimes nicely "packaged" in a quasi-scientific format through a credible- looking speaker. Up to now, there is no scientific proof that food or food supplements can prevent or cure COVID-19 infections (EU, 2021). Moreover, there is no scientific evidence that food is a transmission route or poses a risk for COVID-19 proliferation (EFSA, 2020) because these coronaviruses have poor survivability on surfaces as foodstuffs or packaging (CDC, 2020). However, that has not prevented some companies claiming that their products and brands are safer only because they use automatic packaging equipment and offer pre-packed food. To support their case, they have "fabricated" some pieces of pseudo- scientific evidence. This situation is made worse when the press uncritically repeats and distributes these claims.

News headlines in a European country reported in 2020 about the potential transmission of SARS-CoV-2 through fresh food (bread), encouraging the consumers to eat only pre-packed bread products; dedicated advertising to consume pre-packed bread happened to be offered under a certain brand. Later, advertising with such messages was forbidden because it was considered unfair competition and induced panic among consumers. Besides, it lacks scientific support. However, a few months later, a scientific study on the risks and transmission routes of COVID-19 was initiated on packaged versus unpackaged bread, and surprisingly enough no other food products.

The study was carried out by a team from a well-regarded university, although the team had no specific expertise in food. Consequently, the study remains controversial, with doubts about the methodology, the ethics, and the results. The conclusion was that only unpacked products can be contaminated with COVID-19, the period of viruses' survival on food surfaces being up to 3 h. By packaging in plastic wrap (polyethylene or polypropylene), food products would no longer be exposed to the risk of COVID-19 contamination, as the virus cannot penetrate the packaging material, and food contamination can be avoided.

Not surprisingly, the results were not published in a peer-review journal but only communicated through a press conference (available on YouTube). No conflicts of interest were declared.

Several food specialists have challenged the study and its conclusions, but they did not hold press conferences and did not manage to draw a large audience. In the meantime, a legislative initiative was started to mandate the exclusive sale of bread in pre-packaged form, or through assisted sale. In the end, the proposed new legislation failed to gather enough support, but this apparently well-organized misinformation campaign almost succeeded.

Discussion and key learnings

- Attempts to leverage a pandemic for commercial purposes by implicitly suggesting that "my company's product is safer," without solid peer-reviewed evidence, are unethical, reflect badly on the company involved, and may ultimately undermine consumer confidence in the food industry.
- The University involved should have prevented a study in a high-profile public health case, carried out by people who did not have the appropriate expertise.
- Presenting highly controversial non peer-reviewed conclusions, without addressing potential conflicts of interest, in a press conference, to the apparent benefit of one company, must also be seen as unethical and may ultimately undermine general public confidence in science.

References

- CDC, 2020. Food Safety and Coronavirus Disease 2019 (COVID-19). CDC Newsletter. Available online at: https://www.cdc.gov/foodsafety/newsletter/food-safety-and-Coronavirus.html.
- EFSA, 2020. Coronavirus: No Evidence that Food Is a Source or Transmission Route. EFSA News. Available online at: https://www.efsa.europa.eu/en/news/coronavirus-no-evidence- food-source-or-transmission-route.
- EU, 2021. Consumer Rights. Available online at: https://ec.europa.eu/info/live-work-travel-eu/ consumer-rights-and-complaints/enforcement-consumer-protection/scams-related-covid- 19_en.
- ICPEN, 2021. Consumer Protection Around the World. Available online at: https://icpen.org/ consumer-protection-around-world.

2.4 Risk perception and food safety priorities

In many parts of the world, people sometimes have a strange perception of what food safety is about. This is even true for members of the health professions. I was working as the head of food safety program in an international organization. In this capacity, one day in the 1990s, I visited a developing country to assess its problems and needs. In that country there was a high incidence of foodborne diarrheal diseases, including infant diarrhoea. I was looking forward to having a frank discussion with the public health authorities on possible interventions, such as consumer education on food safety or training of health professionals.

To my surprise, my counterpart, a senior official from the Ministry of Health, told me that one of their urgent food safety problems was the fact that shops were selling expired canned food! While in a properly regulated food system it is certainly illegal to sell canned food beyond the declared expiry date, such an offense has little or hardly any health consequences.
In the years that followed, I confronted many similar situations and raising awareness on what food safety is about and its importance has been a tough battle.

Discussion and key learnings

The issue of food safety and associated health problems was sometimes - and still is - poorly perceived. This is why raising awareness of the importance of food safety has been a long battle.

It took the bovine spongiform encephalopathy (bovine spongiform encephalopathy [BSE] or mad cow disease) crisis in Europe and an outbreak of Escherichia coli O157 in the United States, where four children died from eating contaminated hamburgers, as well as many other crises, for the world to wake up (Motarjemi, 2014).

As a result of these crises, risk management and risk assessment processes have been revised. Today, public health priorities are based on objective scientific criteria and measures such as the burden of foodborne disease, appropriate level of protection, food safety objectives, rather than on the personal perception of risk by health professionals (Motarjemi and Moy, 2014).

The nature and prevalence of foodborne diseases vary according to the regions of the world, the degree of urbanization, industrialization, water and sanitation infrastructure, and food hygiene education of the population. In the country mentioned in this article, the urgent food safety problem was foodborne diarrhoea caused by a wide range of foodborne pathogens associated with food preparation at home or in cottage industries. As such, the training of health professionals and/or persons responsible for food handling or caregivers should have been the priority measure (Käferstein, 2003, Motarjemi et al. 2012).

References

- Käferstein, F.K., 2003. Food safety: the fourth pillar in the strategy to prevent infant diarrhoea. Bull. World Health Organ. 81, 842-843.
- Motarjemi, Y., Moy, G., Todd, E. (Eds.), 2014. Encyclopedia of Food Safety, Risk Analysis. Academic Press, p. 59-151.
- Motarjemi, Y., Moy, G., 2014. Risk analysis: risk management application to biological hazards. In: Motarjemi, Y., Moy, G., Todd, E. (Eds.), Encyclopedia of Food Safety, Risk Analysis. Academic Press, pp. 1037-1063.

- Motarjemi, Y., 2014. Crisis management. In: Motarjemi, Y., Lelieveld, H. (Eds.), Food Safety Management; a Practical Guide for the Food Industry. Academic Press, pp. 1037-1063.
- Motarjemi, Y., Steffen, R., Binder, H., 2012. Preventive strategy against infectious diarrhoea - a holistic approach. Gastroenterology 143, 516-519.

2.5 The rise of food safety: the long walk

I joined the World Health Organization (WHO) in 1980 to head its new Food Safety Program (FOS).

One of my first actions was to pay a courtesy visit to the head of the Diarrheal Disease Program (CDD). The reason was that I strongly believed that the two programmes - FOS and CDD - needed to work closely together to reduce diarrheal morbidity. To my surprise and disappointment, my counterpart in CDD told me that he would not see the point of such cooperation since only contaminated water, not food, was responsible for the onset of diarrhoea! I don't need to say how surprised I was to hear such a point of view. Despite my efforts and all the reasons, this misperception persisted for many years (Moore et al., 2011 and Motarjemi et al., 1993). Together with my team, for many years, I had to fight for the recognition of the role of food in the transmission of diarrheal diseases (Käferstein, 2003; Motarjemi et al., 1993).

At my insistence, after much hesitation, the Director of CDD accepted my proposal to convene a joint scientific consultation of CDD and FOS to determine whether and to what extent contaminated food plays a role in the epidemiology of diarrhoea, including infant diarrhoea of course. The outcome of this consultation became thereafter a reference document for another expert meeting, the FAO/ WHO expert committee on food safety.

In its report, entitled "The Role of Food Safety in Health and Development," the consultation recognized the importance of food in diarrheal diseases and went even further by concluding that "illness due to contaminated food is perhaps the most widespread health problem in the contemporary world and an important cause of reduced economic productivity" (WHO,

1984). This declaration paved the way for the emergence of food safety as a key public health function. A strong program for the prevention and control of foodborne diseases was subsequently put in place. Based on scientific evidence, the role of food in the transmission of childhood diarrhoea as well as other previously neglected diseases such as cholera was recognized (Motarjemi et al., 1993, 2012).

Finally, in 2000, for the first time in its history, the WHO adopted a resolution on food safety and called on WHO Member States to commit themselves to improving food safety.

Discussion and key learnings

Today, the importance of food safety is recognized. However, in order to achieve this, many public health professionals have had to fight against perceived dogmas. Just, as Ignaz Philipp Semmelweis once had to fight to promote handwashing, or before him, Galileo Galilei or other scientists sacrificed their lives to convince society of a scientific truth.

In this story we learn about the efforts that were made to gain recognition for food safety and to encourage public health authorities to pay more attention to this subject. This is all the more important that in the industrial age, where the food chain and the conditions of food production have become more complex, food safety cannot be taken for granted.

Sometimes professionals may also have misperceptions about certain issues, hence the importance of science-based decision-making.

Mankind can accomplish much with perseverance, patience, and integrity. These are the essential characteristics of leadership.

References

- Käferstein, F.K., 2003. Food safety: the fourth pillar in the strategy to prevent infant diarrhoea. Bull. World Health Organ. 81, 842-843.
- Moore, S.R., Lima, A.A., Guerrant, R.L., 2011. Infection: preventing 5 million child deaths from diarrhoea in the next 5 year. Nat. Rev. Gastroenterol. Hepatol. 8, 363-364.
- Motarjemi, Y., Käferstein, F., Moy, G., et al., 1993. Contaminated weaning food: a major risk factor for diarrhoea and associated malnutrition. Bullet. World Health Organ. 71, 79-92.
- Motarjemi, Y., Steffen, R., Binder, H., 2012. Preventive strategy against infectious diarrhoea-a holistic approach. Gastroenterology 143 (3), 516. www.gastrojournal.org/article/S0016-5085(12)01014-1/fulltext.
- WHO, 1984. The role of food safety in health and development. Report of a FAO/WHO Expert Committee on food safety. World Health Organ. Tech. Rep. Ser. 705.

Further reading

WHO, May 20, 2000. Resolution World Health Assembly 53, 15.

2.6 Lessons from a food hygiene training

A food company conducted training for all 700 employees, across their four manufacturing sites, on a yearly basis. They used to hire external experts for this purpose.

One year, I was asked to give a training on the topic "Application of basic hygiene rules." I discussed content and organizational issues with the quality managers beforehand and we decided that I should do exactly the same training at all production sites, although different products were manufactured and different processes were used in each case.

Groups of 25 people were formed by the management, based on availability and in order not to disrupt the workflow as much as possible. For example, cleaning staff, secretaries, technical staff, lab technicians, and production managers could be all in the same group.

Based on the training conducted in previous years, the learning objective and content of my program was precisely defined, as well as which test to take with all participants at the end of a session to measure the learning success. At the request of the management but against my advice, the results of this test were linked to a bonus- malus system for the staff. A session lasted 60 min including the test, and I timed my presentation so that there was enough time for questions and discussion. For efficiency, several training sessions were held on the same day and at the same location.

After the first training session, there was a short discussion with the quality manager, who confirmed that my training had met his expectations and that I should continue in the same way. In all subsequent training sessions, there was no more feedback from my clients. Most of the students said goodbye quickly after a lesson, and only a few discussed what they had heard with me. In such a situation it is impossible for a trainer to improve and adapt his lessons to the needs of the audience.

Discussion and key learnings

The aim of the training was to refresh the knowledge of the employees so that their correct behavior regarding hygiene in practice becomes second nature. It was not the primary aim of the course for them to understand the background to the hygiene rules. Nevertheless, I also strongly emphasized these backgrounds, but because there were groups with participants of very different levels of knowledge and previous education, it was not always easy to keep everybody motivated throughout the lesson.

In such a situation, the best didactic tool is to teach a lot with practical examples and even better with demonstrations. This worked very well in this case by letting the participants do small experiments and showing them the results later. This was very much appreciated because most of the students were machine operators, who preferred learning by doing.

Having a final test at the end of training is good, because you can design it in such a way that it is almost playful and even funny and it provides an additional learning effect. But it is completely wrong to combine the training and the test with a bonus- malus system for the employees, because that creates stress and, for many, the feeling of failure right from the start. At this point, my objectives as a trainer conflicted with the wishes of management.

It is my experience that lessons of 60 min is the maximum that can be expected of production workers in a food factory.

Typically, they are not comfortable sitting still and listening for extended periods of time. If the training is then also scheduled at the end of the working day, it is not surprising to see some dozing off. Equally unfavorable is the time after lunch, and so training sessions in the morning work best. It is important that a spacious room is available and that the technical infrastructure is in place and functioning. In this case that was not always so, although I was assured it would be. As an external trainer, you can try to think of many potential difficulties and suggest possible solutions. The participants associate the technical problems they encounter with the company and not with you as a trainer, and you need to be careful to maintain a positive learning atmosphere and not let discussions deteriorate into company bashing.

Typically, the staff of food companies are multicultural. This aspect is particularly noticeable in the topic of hygiene, but can also be incorporated perfectly into the lessons by discussions in the group. Another challenge is the very different language skills of the students, not only because the language in which the training is conducted is not their mother tongue, but also because they may have only a limited formal education. Tests of practical literacy in some companies have shown that up to 15% of workers had difficulty reading and writing and had therefore a limited capacity to follow presentations. Some companies have organized in-house practical literacy training (an expensive and longer-term program) but in "simple" cases; it is an advantage if the trainer is fluent in several relevant languages, supposing the training groups can be formed according to language competence. Still, the trainer will need to develop a good sense for when they are losing the audience because of language problems.

A disadvantage for external trainers is that they don't know attendees, their functions in the company, their knowledge, concerning the course topic, or their professional and personal environment. At every training session, they will see new faces and have to create a positive learning atmosphere within the first few minutes.

For the trainers, and in my experience, four to five such training sessions a day is the maximum that can be delivered while maintaining effectiveness, motivation, and the ability to motivate others.

Further reading

Motarjemi, Y., Lelieveld, H., 2014. Training and education (Chapter 47). In: Motarjemi, Y., Lelieveld, H. (Eds.), Food Safety Management, A Practical Guide for Food Industry. Elsevier.

2.7 Misinterpretation of foodborne disease surveillance systems

All health education specialists know that education and behavior changes are most effective when carried out at an early stage in life.

During a period in my career in the 1990s, when I was responsible for foodborne disease surveillance and prevention, I worked on the health education of consumers, including school children. I too soon realized that trying to change the behavior of adults, although necessary, was not the most effective and sustainable approach to educating consumers and that it was better to educate children and, through them, their parents. My research also showed that people's resistance to changing their behavior was partly due to their lack of understanding and misperception of the world of microbes. The challenge was to get children to see the invisible world of microbes and to introduce them to the concept of food safety. I hoped that the children would then influence their parents.

So, after years of experience in the subject matter, I decided to write a scientific novel for school children aged 7 to 12. In doing this, I applied all the didactic knowledge I had to make it intriguing. My plan was to focus on the science of microbes and control measures rather than writing food hygiene instructions that should come at a later stage by parents or teachers.

After a lot of work and field-testing the draft with some children, the book was finally finished and published. It was well received by experts in food safety and got good reviews from experts in some scientific and public health sources. "Almost an epidemiological investigation," commented a microbiologist! The book was even adapted to a play for children's theater.

Children also loved it. However, more important than liking the book, the impact on children was remarkable. They would question the practices of their parents. For instance, they would ask: Did you wash your hands before preparing the meal? In one case, a child was taking and eating snow from the street. The mother told him that he should not do this. The child refused and replied: See it is clean, there is no dirt. As soon as mother asked if he remembered the book "Invisible Things," the child dropped the snow.

With this success, I decided to share a free copy with the ministries of education and health of each state in my country and propose an educational program. In the introduction of the covering letter, I stated that "foodborne illnesses are a widespread health problem."

A few weeks later, I received a reply from the doctor supervising school health programs, who rejected my proposal. In his reply, he wrote: "Diseases related to excessive hygiene are a bigger problem than foodborne diseases." He added: "In the last ten years we have only had about 100 outbreaks of foodborne diseases, so they are not as big a health problem."

It is worth noting that in that year, the country's public health authorities reported an annual incidence of over 8000 cases of campylobacter in a population of 8 million people (i.e., over 100 cases/100,000 population). Given the underreporting factor, one can assume that the actual incidence is several times higher: yet campylobacter is only one of several hundred foodborne agents that we need to be concerned about. Shortly after the school doctor's statement, Europe was hit by one of its worst foodborne disease outbreaks, namely the Escherichia coli (O104:H4) outbreak associated with contaminated fenugreek.

Today, 10 years later, as this book is being prepared, the world is hit by one of its worst pandemics, COVID-19. Although COVID-19 is not declared foodborne, nevertheless, the education of children, today's adults, in the science of microbes could have contributed to the management of the crisis and facilitated their education in protective barriers.

Discussion and key learnings

The education of children is important on several counts. First, for their own protection and, as adults, for the protection of their families. However, some may end up working in food establishments or the medical and health profession. In order for good behavior to become ingrained in their minds, it is important to understand the concept of microbes from an early age.

However, the subject of this story is not so much the promotion of education for children, which may be obvious to most readers, but the ignorance of some health professionals about foodborne illness and how they interpret the statistics collected by surveillance systems.

There are different surveillance systems. The number of reported cases varies according to the surveillance methods: outbreak-related surveillance, disease notifications, laboratory-confirmed cases, sentinel surveillance, or population-based surveillance.

Cases of foodborne disease related to outbreaks are only a small fraction of the actual incidence of foodborne diseases, i.e., the tip of the iceberg. The figure illustrates the difference in data in the Netherlands depending on the surveillance system (Motarjemi et al., 2012; Borgdorff and Motarjemi, 1997).

The reasons for these differences are diverse. As another story in this book points out (see story 3.15 Fish soup intoxication: where is the investigation?), people suffering from a foodborne illness do not always consult a doctor and the medical personnel do not report self-limiting illnesses. In addition, there is no official surveillance system for all foodborne diseases. Much also depends on the nature and severity of the illness. The best data are obtained through active epidemiological research, such as a population-based survey.

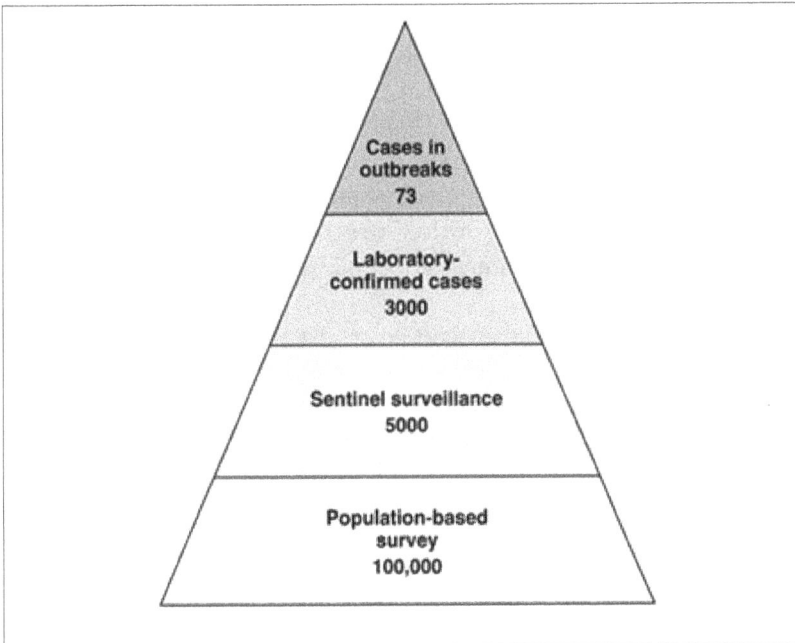

The importance of interpretation of data (salmonellosis in The Netherlands in 1991-1994) in considering the outcome of the different systems of surveillance. Adapted from Borgdorff MW and Motarjemi Y. Surveillance of Foodborne Diseases: What are the Options? WHO Document: WHO/FSF/ FOS/97.31997, World Health Organization, Geneva, 1997. Original figure is adapted from P. Sockett, PhD thesis (Motarjemi, 2012).

References

- Borgdorff, M., Motarjemi, Y., 1997. Surveillance of foodborne diseases: what are the options? World Health Statis. Quarter. 50 (1/2).
- Motarjemi, Y., Steffen, R., Binder, H.J., 2012. Preventive strategy against infectious diarrhoea–a holistic approach. Gastroenterology 143 (3), 516-519.

Further reading

- EFSA, 2011. Tracing Seeds, in Particular Fenugreek (Trigonella goenum-graecum) Seeds, in Relation to the Shiga Toxin-Producing E. coli (STEC) O104:H4 2011 Outbreaks in Germany and France. Technical Report of EFSA. EFSA, Parma, Italy.
- Motarjemi, Y., 2011. Food safety: what is the role for gastroenterologists? World Gastroenterol. News 16 (3). https://www.worldgastroenterology.org/UserFiles/file/e-wgn/e-wgn-2011-september.pdf.
- OFSP.   Campylobactériose: https://www.bag.admin.ch/bag/fr/home/krankheiten/krankheiten-   im-ueberblick/campylobacteriose.html.
- WHO, 1997. Surveillance of Foodborne Diseases: What Are the Options? (WHO Document WHO/FSF/FOS/97.3). World Health Organization, Geneva, Switzerland. https://apps. who.int/iris/handle/10665/63479
- WHO/Euro. Outbreaks of E. coli O104:H4 infection: update 30. https://www.euro.who.int/en/ health-topics/disease-prevention/food-safety/news/news/2011/07/outbreaks-of-e.-coli-   o104h4-infection-update-30.

2.8 The human factor in food safety

I didn't know, forgot; couldn't or chose not to.

For decades I have worked around the world training, implementing, and troubleshooting food safety systems and standards. There are many stories to tell over those years. Here's one that sums up human behavior.

Ten years ago, a foodborne intoxication outbreak occurred at a hotel on a famous tourist site. A large number of adolescents were affected. Together with other experts and inspectors, we were engaged to investigate the outbreak. Very quickly, we found that on that day and the day before, the adolescents had eaten at three different restaurants.

In the first restaurant, Escherichia coli and large number of coliforms were found on the kitchen surfaces. In the second, the same microorganisms were found in the mixer. In the third restaurant, nothing wrong was found. However, it was reported that some kids had been drinking water from a fountain near the third restaurant. Next to the fountain, a sign had been placed by the state authority, telling people that the water from the fountain is not potable, but at the time, the sign was missing.

We also interviewed the restaurant personnel about their practices. The cook in the first restaurant stated that he was angry with his boss, because the boss demanded regular cleaning and disinfection, but the cook was not always provided with cleaning agents and disinfectants and he was tired of buying them out of his own pocket. Also, nobody ever checked whether the kitchen was clean or not. So, he decided that he would not clean the kitchen until the day he received the necessary materials. Also, he said that the second shift cook (who was the chef) chose not to clean at all because he thought that it was not his job, so why should he (the cook in the first shift) be solely held responsible, or do it if his boss did not do it.

In the second restaurant, the cook stated that he received a training course in food hygiene long ago, but the training was confusing. So, he did not know whether he was cleaning properly. He also said that during the off-season, a lot of staff had been laid off. Consequently, not only was he the only cook in the restaurant, but he also had the duty of purchasing raw materials, transporting food to other small restaurants as caterer, do all the cleaning, and much more. Having all of these tasks, he simply forgot to clean that day.

Regarding the sign, it was found that the employees from the third restaurant removed the warning sign next to the water fountain, because they thought that the sign which was placed a few meters from their restaurant was scaring people, and that this was the main reason why they had less clients than expected.

Discussion and key learnings

Human errors can be classified into four major categories: (1) I didn't know; (2) I forgot; (3) I couldn't; and (4) I chose not to. Although often intertwining, in general, a different explanation can be given for each of them.

For the category "I didn't know," the usual reason is a lack of adequate training. The responsibility for training is with the company owner and/or Quality Assurance team. Sometimes, the language or the techniques of training are not adapted to the audience and the training is far too complicated for the trainees to understand and learn. Sometimes, there is a lack of definition of responsibilities and the employee may not know that a given task is his/her responsibility.

For the category "I forgot," the explanation is much simpler. It is based on lack of the awareness of the importance of the subject. Food businesses have to establish an awareness plan, including training and refresher training, posting signs and posters, staff briefings, awareness boards, etc. Work overload may also be a reason for forgetting.

The category "I couldn't" generally has two origins: lack of skills, that is, there was no qualified person for the assigned task, or the person responsible is overloaded and there is no one to support him/her. Lack of resources such as personnel, equipment, tools, materials, and specifications can also be the reason. Responsibility for this lays equally with food company owners and/or purchasing personnel.

The last category "I'm angry with my organization" is the most dangerous, because it usually points to intentional noncompliance, or in other terms a violation related to internal company tensions. There are several subcategories for this behavior. People are angry with their boss because they feel undercompensated, or they are angry with their superiors who do not seem to care about or respect the employee. When employees are saying "I do not see why I have to do it," it means that their shift leaders and supervisors should "walk the talk" or, more precisely, should do what they preach. The feeling of "nobody cares" drives to noncompliance. Employees need to know that their work is monitored and important and good work is appreciated. Similarly, the claim "Why should I care?" means that there is lack of commitment, laziness, and wrong attitude, or pure malice.

When we are speaking about ensuring food safety, we are aiming to act on the risk factors and reduce risks to an "as low as reasonably achievable" level (ALARA concept). In this context, human behavior is one of the key risk factors that should be addressed. So far, all the attention is focused on biological and toxicological sciences and studying hazards, be it microbiological, chemical, allergens, physical, or establishing the rules and procedures for food hygiene, such as cleaning, testing, and processing. However, according to my experience, in 95% of the cases, the main reason for foodborne illness incidents is human behavior. It is time for human behavior to receive specific attention in the systems of food safety management and investigation of outbreaks.

Further reading

- Kakurinov, V., 2017. Human behavior - 4th hazard in food safety. J. Hygi. Eng. Design 21, 13-17.
- Motarjemi, Y., 2014. Chapter 37 - Human factors in food safety management. In: Motarjemi, Y., Lelieveld, H. (Eds.), Food Safety Management. A Practical Guide for the Food Industry, pp. 975-986.

Chapter Three

Incident investigations and management

3.1 Ice cream: contaminated product destruction

The company I worked for produced ice cream, under the brand name of a major retailer. Part of the contractual obligations was that batches be delivered accompanied by a certificate of analysis, which, among others, included a total viable count (TVC) number. The specification included an upper limit for TVC.

One day, the lab reported that they found the TVC number to be over the limit. There was only one conclusion for this batch: it had to be destroyed. In this case the product was considered to be still good enough as pig feed and a large pig farmer was contracted for this job. As per company procedure, one of the Quality Assurance (QA) people went with the frozen truck to the pig farm, in order to witness the destruction - on a Friday. At the farm, workers had to unpack the product and remove all primary packaging material, which then had to be collected and destroyed separately. Everything seemed to be going well, but this batch was rather large and by Friday 6 p.m., the job was not finished yet. It was agreed that work would continue during the evening hours, because there was no refrigeration capacity at the farm and leaving the product overnight - or even over the weekend - at ambient temperatures would create a mess. The company QA man felt that everything was clearly agreed and understood and that it was time for him to go home.

As soon as he left, the workers decided that the destruction of what appeared to be perfectly good looking and smelling ice cream - and a premium brand too - was an incomprehensible and unnecessary waste. They started calling friends and relatives at the village nearby and people came to the farm, loaded their trunks full of litre packs of this delicious product, and shared that among neighbors and everybody who wanted a pack or two.

Then, on Saturday morning, a lady felt this was too good to be true and she called the service line of the retailer, informing them that free litre packs of their ice cream were being handed out all over the village. Could the retailer tell her what this was all about? The retailer could not. They had not been informed, but proceeded to call the producing company. An immediate public recall was the only possible outcome, but this was a special case. Distribution was - we could safely assume - restricted to one village only and we could not afford to wait until the normal channels (newspapers mainly) would reach the villagers. Furthermore, we could also assume that a very large percentage of the households actually had a pack in their possession.

We called the mayor, explained the situation, got his support, and on Sunday morning representatives of the company went door to door to explain and retrieve product. In the meantime, word got out and a photographer from the largest national newspaper followed the recall.

People in the whole country saw the pictures on Monday. Nobody got sick, as far as we know.

Discussion and key learnings

Three major mistakes had been made here: (1) the destruction was supposed to be witnessed, but in the end, it was not and control was lost, (2) it was not sufficiently explained to the workers at the pig farm that this product was no longer fit for human consumption, never mind how good it looked and smelled, and (3) the customer - the retailer - was not informed.

They were extremely annoyed about this episode and insisted on tightened procedures - on top of an investigation into the cause of the out-of-spec TVC.

Further reading

Overbosch, P., Carter, J.C., 2014. Food safety assurance systems: recall systems and disposal of food. Encyclopedia of Food Safety. Academic Press, Waltham, Massachusetts, pp. 309-314.

3.2 Syringe in ice cream

An ice cream producing company in an Eastern European country received a consumer complaint. A part of a needle of a syringe had been found in an ice cream that a family had for dessert, but only after it got stuck in the roof of a young boy's mouth. The father of the boy happened to be a medical doctor and at that particular evening there was a guest at the table, a lawyer. They wanted an apology, compensation, and an explanation.

The family was not willing to hand over the needle, as they felt this was the physical proof of what had happened and they wanted to hold onto it, but they were willing to show the object to representatives of the company, who wanted to see it for investigative purposes. All sides agreed that this was indeed a part of a syringe needle and internal investigations in the company confirmed that no such syringe was in use for any purpose at the production line or belonged to the maintenance toolkit. It had to have been brought in from the outside, probably specifically for tampering purposes. The question where it had entered the product was easier, it could only have been introduced right before packaging - there was no good opportunity to do it earlier, and anyway the processing steps would probably have broken the needle into much smaller fragments. The conclusion at that stage was that this was a case of malicious tampering, with the intention of harming a consumer - and probably by implication also the company, or vice versa.

The investigators could not help but think that having the object end up in a little boy's mouth, with a doctor and a lawyer present, was probably just the kind of damage the perpetrator had been aiming for.

The next question was how the needle could have passed the metal detectors at the end of the line. An object of similar shape and size was introduced in a specially marked package, and it passed. This was clearly not what the company had expected, and they continued to investigate. The normal routine for checking the metal detector's effectiveness - before each production run - involved passing a single package through the detector, loaded with a standard metal object. During actual production, units of six packs ran through the detector, and that made a significant difference in the effective sensitivity of the detector. Furthermore, the orientation of the needle in the product mattered. If it was oriented parallel to the direction of the conveyor belt, in six packs, it was detected some of the time, but if oriented perpendicular to the belt, it was not. The company finally decided to run single products only through two metal detectors, placed at an angle to each other. The boy suffered no lasting consequences, and the family did receive an apology, an explanation, and some compensation. The perpetrator was never found, but the episode did not repeat itself.

Discussion and key learnings

- Malicious tampering happens - and this author has seen a number of cases. Physically protecting the product as much as possible is always worthwhile, but the problem may never entirely disappear.
- A routine check on the effectiveness of a metal detector is normal practice, but the check should be carried out under the exact same conditions as normal production runs (in the case, six packs vs. single pack).

3.3 What if your customer becomes a threat?

In the first years of this millennium, the food industry was tormented by the bovine spongiform encephalopathy (BSE) crisis. The BSE outbreak caused severe economic and reputation damage to the meat industry and led to serious health concerns for authorities and consumers. One of the measures taken in the European Union (EU) was to establish an extensive laboratory test program; all slaughtered cattle older than 30 months needed to be examined for the presence of BSE prions.

In the Netherlands alone, more than 500,000 slaughtered cows per year needed to be tested for BSE. High demands were placed on speed, traceability, and quality of sampling and testing. Within 2 months, a testing program was set up by the government. In the Netherlands, all routine BSE screening was set up and carried out by the Central Institute for Animal Disease and Control (CIDC) in Lelystad. Once the program was up and running, there was growing market pressure to outsource testing to private laboratories. Companies expected to get a higher service level and lower prices and referred to other EU countries where lab tests were done by private laboratories.

After much hesitation, the Dutch government decided to outsource BSE testing to a few licensed laboratories in the private sector but under supervision of the CIDC. The CIDC implemented and maintained a solid control regime and kept end responsibility of the BSE monitoring in the Netherlands. This control regime included weekly unannounced expert audits. The main reasons for these strict policies were food safety and economical (export) concerns and a lack of trust regarding the meat industry in general.

At that point in time, I was working as a lab manager in one of the licensed laboratories entering the BSE testing market. We quickly discovered that working for slaughterhouses is different than working for - let's say - the convenience food industry. Slaughterers can be quite persistent, persuasive, impatient, and bullying if things do not go their way. Also, we were pretty annoyed by the weekly governmental audits and corresponding demands plus extra workload. But in the end, things settled down and we found our way in the world of BSE testing.

One day our sales manager brought in a big new customer; a slaughterhouse restarting after bankruptcy. From the beginning on, we had a lot of complaints regarding unfit samples. A BSE test needs to be performed on a sample from the obex region of the brainstem because this part has the highest concentration of BSE particles (prions). A sample with a damaged or unrecognizable obex is considered an unfit sample. Unfit samples can and must still be tested, but if the result is negative (no prions detected), it is reported as indecisive.

An indecisive result has a huge impact, the carcass concerned needs to be destroyed, and also complete batches of fat, blood, and other materials that might have been contaminated should be treated as high-risk waste. So instead of making money out of these products, the slaughterhouse was incurring a significant increase in cost.

We tested about 800 to 1000 brainstems per week and normally we had one or two unfit samples per 6 months. With this particular customer we had 10 per week during the start-up month. Did I already mention that slaughterhouse staff can be impatient, bullying, etc.? Of course, the lab is to blame, although we serviced many similar customers without similar issues.

So, I had a 200 km drive in the middle of the night to have a look at the slaughter process at the site. The slaughterhouse director and veterinarian (who did the sampling) joined me during this audit. Quickly I found that the way the slaughtered animals were skinned was causing damage to the brainstem and I did some recommendations for improvement. My thoughts were "Problem solved, happy customer and back to the lab," but the "fun" part still had to begin.

We gathered at the director's office and the director said: "Okay gentlemen, let us agree that from this moment on we will never again have an unfit sample at this slaughterhouse." The vet and I both replied that we could not guarantee this. He walked over to me, glared me in the eye, and repeated his statement. On my second refusal, he prodded his finger in my chest and said empathically, "Kiddo, mark my words, you will never ever report an unfit sample again." Hmm "kiddo?" I was in my forties and had never such an experience since high school.

In the end he cooled down a little and seemed sensitive to the argument that besides our own quality management system we were under strict government control. But his box of tricks was not exhausted yet and he suggested to replace any unfit sample with new brainstems from freshly slaughtered calves. So, I could still do the test but on a sample that surely was going to give a negative test result. He was not receptive to my reply that this would be fraud. "There is no BSE problem in the Netherlands so switching brainstems has no food safety consequences, end of discussion." I did not give in to him but his last words when I left were: "Remember kiddo, no more unfit samples." Funny how some words keep resonating in your head.

Fortunately, we did not find any unfit samples from this slaughterhouse anymore, so no more nocturnal trips and difficult discussions.

One year later, the slaughterhouse filed for bankruptcy.

Discussion and key learnings

Although most private laboratories have a good quality system, you need to protect your staff against improper pressure and demands from customers. It should be incorporated in your written and unwritten procedures and addressed during training. I was lucky because of my age and experience in customer contact roles. Besides this I knew that I was backed and covered by my manager.

Although the governmental supervision program was another safeguard for me during this incident, I think such a program is an overkill, adding unnecessary cost and another external pressure to your staff.

Of course, we researched the market segment of the meat industry before entering that market, but this research was more about opportunities, turnover, and profit and not so much about risks due to improper customer pressure. Although this slaughterhouse was an exception, I think it is wise to incorporate the subject of inappropriate customer pressure in your research and include suitable integrity measures in your procedures and training modules. Make sure that your staff knows they are supported by their company.

Also be aware that the majority of laboratory staff have little or no experience with direct customer contact.

Even if you are not entering a new market segment, existing customers can be under big (financial) pressure and might start acting similar to the way the director of the slaughterhouse. So, prepare your management and staff.

Take extra care if it concerns "big" customers with substantial turnover. In this example the slaughterhouse was good for 40% of BSE turnover.

3.4 Penicillium roqueforti in cans

The product for discussion in this story was an intermediate moisture food, packaged in a can. Vegetative organisms were controlled via pasteurization of the sealed cans. Spore-forming bacteria were controlled by the low water activity which prevented their outgrowth. The product had a relatively long history without issues.

This incident began when the company began to get some disturbing consumer complaints. Consumers were calling to say that the product smelled of gasoline, kerosene, or other harmful chemicals, and they were frightened that it had been tampered with. Isolated complaints of this nature were received over a period of months.

All of the consumers involved had used some of the product at an earlier date and said that they were worried that they might have exposed their families and themselves to a harmful chemical. None of the consumers had experienced any symptoms related to consumption of the product but they were nervous. None of the consumers had consumed the product once they detected the odor.

Some of the consumers contacted their local Health Department at the same time as they complained to the company, but as the containers had been opened for some time, there were not multiple complaints related to one batch, and the retention samples at the production facility were normal, the Health Department did not pursue with urgency.

However, the company felt there was a cause for concern. The consumers that had been in contact were loyal product users and seemed genuinely concerned. Additionally, as a company, it was important to determine the root cause.

When the first complaint came in, the sample was collected from the consumer and was indeed found to exhibit a strong petrochemical smell. The company considered it a very serious matter as there was the potential that the product had been tampered with - somewhere in the distribution chain after production - even though it was sold in a sealed can. As the first complaint was being analyzed, another complaint was received which escalated the situation. There did not seem to be any connection between the consumers, the retailers, or the actual batches of production.

The fear that the company was dealing with a tampering incident increased, although the typical signs of malicious tampering - threats or ransom notes, geographical clustering of the incidents, visible damage of the can (punctures) - were absent.

The internal investigation was given the highest priority. Concurrent investigations were carried out. Seals on the cans were tested, and retention samples from the factory were analyzed along with the consumer samples. The product was produced in a small can as well as a newer consumer unit in a large can. The complaints received were all from the larger can, so product heating profiles were compared, and plant data were analyzed to see if there was any difference. The raw materials were also tested.

The samples were tested for microbiological and chemical contaminants. Gasoline and kerosene were not detected and many other contaminants were not found; however, the chemical analysis of the consumer complaint products revealed that the samples contained 1,3-pentadiene. At the same time, microbiological testing isolated Penicillium roqueforti. These results pointed not to tampering, but to a much less sinister explanation.

Discussion and key learnings

As is often the case, several factors led to the conditions needed to create the issue. The situation was actually a spoilage incident. The product contained sorbic acid which was added to preserve it after opening by the consumer. P. roqueforti is capable of degrading sorbic acid and 1,3-pentadiene is a compound formed through the decarboxylation of sorbic acid. 1,3-Pentadiene has a strong petrochemical odor. In addition, the introduction of a larger can meant that consumers opened the can and kept it around the house for longer periods of time, thus providing more time for the product to pick up the common mold spores and grow to a level where the chemical was produced.

This was an interesting case study as it initially appeared to be a potentially very serious food safety tampering issue. Whereas it was eventually discovered to be a spoilage by-product formed as the result of slow degradation of sorbic acid by a common household mold. The company solution was to eliminate the larger can offering as well as label the smaller cans with clear consumer advice to keep refrigerated after opening and discard after 3 weeks. Once this was done, the company did not have any further issues.

3.5 Allergen ignorance

The corporate consumer contact department takes a toll-free call one afternoon where the caller claims to have had an anaphylactic reaction after eating the company's brand of chocolate ice cream and has recovered. The person states that he has a severe peanut allergy. While there are no other complaints about peanuts or allergic reactions, there is an immediate need for a thorough investigation.

The company has a major brand and a very large distribution area. If this isn't a mistaken claim, the results could be deadly. A team of professional food safety experts was sent to the producing location that same day to determine what had happened. How could peanuts get into a plain chocolate ice cream? They did not have any peanuts in the location. After reviewing records and interviewing production employees, it was discovered that chocolate ice cream frequently contained rework from other flavors, including chocolate peanut butter flavor! They did not understand the allergen risk from peanut butter and other nuts, etc. Allergen awareness was completely lacking.

A total recall of all the company's chocolate ice cream in distribution commenced along with television and print warnings put out to destroy any of the chocolate ice cream in consumer's freezers.

Discussion and key learnings

Control of allergens in food manufacturing is deadly serious. A product that contains an unlabelled allergen could lead to an extremely serious allergic reaction in certain people. In this case the company quickly developed an allergen training program that included creation of plant allergen control plans for allergen storage, equipment separation, dedicated allergen hand tools, and sanitation protocols. These included tests such as adenosine triphosphate (ATP) and enzyme-linked immunosorbent assay (ELISA) that can be used to verify adequate cleaning of common equipment for both allergen and nonallergen containing product.

One important precaution not involved in this case but still an important control factor is label control. Packaging can be very similar. Chocolate ice cream and chocolate peanut butter ice cream printed packaging might look essentially the same with only print and ingredient lines differentiating the two different types. Human error can mix the packaging on the line or in storage. By mistake, the two types of packaging material may be mixed up somewhere on the line or in storage.

Regular line label checks should be in place and recorded. In addition, bar code scanners can be used to detect when an incorrect package is used. In any case, this is a risk that must be managed.

The key to all of this is a well-educated work force in the importance of allergen control.

Further reading

- US Food and Drug Administration (FDA). Appendix 10. Cleaning and Sanitation for the Control of Allergens. https://www.fda.gov/media/129671/download.
- SQFI Guidance RE: 2.8.3 Allergen Cleaning and Sanitation. https://www.sqfi.com/wp-content/uploads/2018/08/Allergen-Guidance-Document.pdf.

3.6 Baby food and a failure in the sterilization process

One day we received several complaints from consumers, claiming that baby food sold in jars had a strange smell and taste. In other words, they were rotten. Immediately after confirming the issue, our operating company issued a product recall.

The investigation showed that a batch of the product had left the plant without having been sterilized. The product batch was caught between two shifts and the change in personnel. The new worker of the new shift had, mistakenly, concluded that baskets of product awaiting sterilization had already been processed.

To our surprise, we learned that the factory's quality manager had been aware of the problem, but reported it only when the product was already on the market and first complaints were coming in.

When questioned, she indicated that she was aware of a spoilage risk, but not of any food safety risk. Her idea was that if the product was not (yet) noticeably spoiled by the time it was served, nobody would notice and no harm would be done. If, on the other hand, it was clearly spoiled by that time, the product would smell bad and parents would not give it to their child, and also in that case no harm would be done.

Discussion and key learnings

Manufacturing sites for retorted products need to be divided into a "raw" and a "processed" side, where the only way to get from one side to the other is through the retort. If no physical barrier exists, mistakes like this will inevitably happen (and they have happened more than once at various sites). If a barrier does exist, operations can be handed from one shift to the next without problems.

What made matters worse is that the plant's quality manager obviously did not understand the significance of the sterilization process being a Critical Control Point in the Hazard Analysis and Critical Control Point (HACCP) plan, meaning that this sterilization step must be carried out correctly in order to assure the safety of the product. Also, she did not realize that the product may present safety risks without necessarily smelling or tasting bad. For instance, baby food in jars present the potential risk of botulinum toxin; therefore, it needs to undergo a "botulinum cook" in the retort. Understanding HACCP principles and food safety hazards and risks is a basic professional requirement for Quality Assurance/Food Safety (QA/FS) management, of which the plant quality manager apparently was unaware.

Finally, she did not report the incident and hoped that the problem could go unnoticed. Irrespective of a professional understanding of the risks involved, not reporting the release of a defective product (not appropriately processed) must count as a dereliction of duty by a QA/FS manager.

In other cases, QA/FS managers have been under pressure to avoid recalls which may (or may not) have been a factor here.

Further reading

- Wareing, P., 2017. Controlling Clostridium botulinum e Using challenge testing to create safe chilled foods. A Leatherhead Food Research white paper. https://www.leatherheadfood. com/files/2017/04/White-paper-45-Controlling-Clostridium-botulinum.pdf.

- Motarjemi, Y., 2014. Human factors in food safety management. In: Motarjemi, Y., Lelieveld, H. (Eds.), Food Safety Management: A Practical Guide for the Food Industry. Academic Press, Waltham, MA, pp. 975-986.
- Motarjemi, Y., Wallace, C., 2014. Incident management and root cause analysis. In: Motarjemi, Y., Lelieveld, H. (Eds.), Food Safety Management: A Practical Guide for the Food Industry. Academic Press, Waltham, MA, pp. 1017-1036.

3.7 A botulism outbreak at Christmas

It was the day after Christmas when the head of the official food control of our region called me at home to inform me that 12 consumers with suspected botulism had been admitted to the nearest university hospital and were being ventilated there. He asked me to come to him and informed me of what was known so far. All 12 people worked at the same company and were also present at the party the company organized for its employees 2 days before Christmas to end the year. As usual at such occasions, wine and beer were served; cold snacks were eaten with cheese, cured meat products, olives, mixed pickles, and similar finger food. In addition, many people still smoked at that time.

All 12 patients consulted the same doctor, who was on emergency duty over the holidays, on 24 or 25 December, complaining of nausea, headaches, and vomiting. This doctor suspected that it might be a more serious problem and phoned a colleague at the university hospital, who raised the suspicion of botulism. In the blood samples taken, antibodies against botulin type B were detected in all 12 patients and they were hospitalized immediately.

My colleague showed me a raw cured ham that could possibly be the cause of the diseases. We cut off a piece and noticed a faint putrid smell and that the central parts were grey and did not show any typical curing color. Later, the neurotoxin type B was detected in this ham. A bacteriological analysis of the ham was not carried out.

Discussion and key learnings

The raw ham could be identified without doubt as the cause of this botulism outbreak before Christmas. Clostridium botulinum or its spores were able to penetrate the inner zones of the ham along the boundary between the muscle tissue and the fat layer and multiply there during processing, especially during salting and the first phase of drying, and form toxin, because the curing salt, especially the nitrite, did not reach the central parts. As this type of product is always eaten raw, toxin formation was ultimately not inactivated before consumption. This was visible as there was no typical pink curing color there. Good production practice for cured ham in small- and medium-sized enterprises is based on many years of experience, but there is no known effective way for them to ascertain that effective curing has taken place down to central zones for all products. A check on correct curing is carried out by cutting open individual pieces of a batch and inspecting them. This procedure typically provides a good indication of the effectiveness of the curing process, but it does not quite rise to the HACCP requirement of assuring that hazards have been eliminated or reduced to an acceptable level. As a result, the producer of the ham shipped his product in good faith, but did not know that one piece of his production posed a great danger to the health of consumers. Only the person who cut and sliced the ham immediately before the party started could have seen and smelled that this ham was not sufficiently cured and should not have been served.

In terms of HACCP, there is a major problem here. The HACCP plan at the producer needs to assure that all product shipped is unconditionally safe, but the standard curing operation may not always be fully effective, and the sampling/cutting checks may not always reveal the problem if there is one. By design, therefore, this product is not sufficiently safe. In practice, the final control point then lies with the customer, which is less than acceptable from a HACCP point of view and also unlikely to be effective, because in this case the putrid smell was faint and dissipated quickly after slicing. Furthermore, the party atmosphere, swarmed with alcohol and smoke, was not conducive to sharpening attention.

The patients were very lucky for two reasons. First, the concentration of the toxin was very low and the amount of ham consumed was small. Secondly, because of the holidays, they all consulted the same doctor, who fortunately brought the 12 cases together and made the correct diagnosis. Foodborne botulism cases are often not recognized or misdiagnosed because the first symptoms are not typical for botulism. In this case, all patients could be discharged from the hospital after a few days to weeks in good health. However, the company producing the ham was closed.

Further reading

Peck, M.W., 2014. Clostridium botulinum. In: Motarjemi, Y., Moy, G., Todd, E. (Eds.), Encyclopaedia of Food Safety, 3. Academic Press, Waltham, Massachusetts, pp. 381-394.

3.8 Fruit juice spoilage

A company in Latin America was marketing ready-to-drink fruit juice in brick presentation. Half of the production was done in-house and the other half at a co-manufacturer. The co-manufacturer was an established company specialized in juice production, properly approved by company auditors, and following mutually agreed food safety and process control standards. Production and sales were running well, in fact above expectations.

Then, consumer complaints started flowing in from several locations, referring to swollen bricks and off-flavored product. The company reacted by checking stock in its warehouses to detect any swelling, while at the same time planning for microtesting of returned samples. It was found that the issue corresponded to the co-manufacturer's product and that it was caused by several, non-pathogenic, spoilage microorganisms. A first review of production records by the co-manufacturer suggested no operational errors, but product was immediately put on hold in all warehouses as a precaution. Production was stopped, and a trade withdrawal was organized.

Stopping production at the co-manufacturer resulted in a subsequent reduction of consumer complaints to pre-event level. However, no specific cause could be identified from microtesting; therefore, a new on-site audit was conducted to better understand causes, as a minimum requirement before authorizing the restart of production.

The on-site audit revealed that in fact there were failures:

- Pasteurization time below agreed HACCP plan.
- Insufficient sanitizer speed in equipment during cleaning-

in-place operations, which left some visible solid residues in certain parts of the equipment.
- Gaps in temperature records (thermograph).
- Diversion valve position not recorded continuously.
- Inconsistent temperature controls of fresh fruit.

While the co-manufacturer worked to address these issues, they requested to manage the withdrawal process in order to guarantee quarantine and destruction at a remote location under their control. After some weeks, the company started receiving again complaints of swollen bricks and off-flavored product. Investigations revealed that complaints were coming from the geographical area where product on hold was being destroyed. What happened is that locals were curious about product in apparently good state being destroyed and took some for their own consumption. The company decided then to stop the destruction by the co-manufacturer, initiated a public recall, and completed the operation under their own supervision at another location. Fortunately, no illness incidents were registered.

As a result of this series of incidents, all production was brought in-house. The co-manufacturing contract was discontinued and a sizable legal negotiation started around the impact of this episode to the brand and business.

Discussion and key learnings

This case shows the importance of day-to-day manufacturing controls and internal verification protocols before releasing product to the market, as opposed to just periodical audits. This is especially critical when it comes to food safety. The co-manufacturer, a well-established company, had in fact been audited and approved, but it still failed to stick to agreed standards. The company was itself not sufficiently organized to monitor the adherence to standards of what was being produced.

Once a product that is manufactured out of specification is released, it is too late to try to sort good from bad based on microtesting - many have tried and have come to regret it. And not all product can be recovered from the market because consumers may not hear about the recall, may just throw the product to the trash, or may have consumed it already.

This case also shows the criticality of robust hold and release procedures when it comes to contain a food safety or quality issue. The co-manufacturer acted in good faith when taking responsibility for the destruction of withdrawn product but failed to control access to the destruction operation and to sufficiently instruct their personnel of potential health risks if products destined for destruction were consumed after all. Food safety issues can destroy a business. In this case, the relationship with the co-manufacturer was terminated, but the negative impact in the form of loss of sales and damage to brand image could not be undone. In the end, the company lost interest in the brand and juice business as a whole and sold the operation.

Further reading

Overbosch, P., Carter, J.C., 2014. Food safety assurance systems: recall systems and disposal of food. In: Encyclopedia of Food Safety. Academic Press, Waltham, MA, pp. 309-314.

3.9 Managing the safety of cheese made with raw milk

I remember where I was when I received the call - in the car park at an external training center, just about to deliver a group presentation to senior leadership peers. You know the kind of thing: "how to improve cross-functional communication" or something similar. The kind of thing that is important to establish your reputation in an organization. Important, but perhaps not urgent.

In food safety and quality, we are always ready for the call. In this case, one of our regional directors had some news - we had been conducting routine randomized testing of private label products in our markets, and a hard cheese product in one of our countries had tested positive for Escherichia coli, commonly known as E. coli.

At my company, this kind of testing was part of the procedure. As a wholesaler/ retailer with close to 2000 private-label manufacturers globally, it was simply not feasible to have direct oversight of all our production sites. So, quality and food safety had to be assured via a robust adherence to the principles of the Global Food Safety Initiative (GFSI) and additional controls to keep our suppliers honest. Trust, but verify.

Testing products for E. coli is a convenient way of assessing the hygiene in a facility. There was no need to panic. Most E. coli species are harmless and indeed these harmless strains are an integral part of the gut flora in humans and other mammals including cattle. But as the organism is common in fecal matter, it is an effective indicator for the good manufacturing practice status of a factory. A positive analytical result in hard cheese, taken from the shelf, confirming the presence of E. coli is not good, although, at times, we had no indication of an imminent or confirmed safety threat.

What should we do? At my company, we had the ability to track exactly who had bought the item (each card purchase is traceable). So, regarding the market action, in principle, there were three options:

1. Leave the product on the market until there were further data on the safety of the products.
2. Remove the product from the shelves without expressively notifying the customers on the issue.
3. Remove from the shelves and perform a recall, contacting customers and the authorities.

At this stage, remember, the only information we had was of a possible hygiene issue at the factory. Nevertheless, as a precautionary measure, the Incident Management Team decided on option 3, and we activated the machinery to withdraw and retrieve the product.

In addition to the market activity, we had to decide what technical steps to take. Of course, we needed to perform an urgent audit at the manufacturing site to focus on improving hygiene, but in addition, did we need to conduct any further testing?

There are two contrasting schools of thought for this testing decision. In one, since the recall decision was already made, there was no need for further information. In the second, a deeper investigation would help us identify the root cause and also be the basis for a legal case with our supplier.

We elected to start an additional analysis.

It is worth mentioning at this point that the product was made with unpasteurized milk.

By this time, of course, I had moved from the car park of the training center. The decisions described so far had taken place over a business day. The recall was initiated, with appropriate (reactive) communications materials saying something like, "in the course of routine testing of our portfolio, our company had identified a quality non-compliance with a specific product (traceability details), and as a precaution we are retrieving from the market and offering relevant compensation."

Also, it is very important to be truthful in these statements. There was a temptation to state that the cheese was completely safe, but as yet we were unable to confirm this.

The analysis had started.

Almost 2 days later, we received the result.

The product was positive for E. coli O157:H7, a dangerous pathogen. Wow.

I had not been expecting this. I had seriously thought that our actions had been cautious and conservative, and I was fully expecting a confirmation of the presence of one or more of the harmless strains mentioned earlier.

Please allow me to quote from Wikipedia here:

> Escherichia coli O157:H7 is one of the Shiga-like toxin producing types of E. coli. It is a cause of disease, typically foodborne illness, through consumption of contaminated and raw food, including raw milk.

Infection with this type of pathogenic bacteria may lead to haemorrhagic diarrhoea, and to kidney failure; these have been reported to cause the deaths of children younger than five years of age, of elderly patients, and of patients whose immune systems are otherwise compromised.

Information like this sharpens the mind. This issue was transformed from a hygiene issue at a factory to potentially a major public food safety incident. Immediately, the Incident Management Team convened and asked ourselves: Have we done enough? Have our customers done enough? And, most importantly, how do we assure that no-one gets sick or worse. We were confident with the actions that we had taken on the market. We had no indication that there were any consumer illnesses, any complaints, or any media report. Definitely, no food safety issue was reported. As mentioned, the strength of the company's business model meant that we were able to contact all customers who had purchased the product and we were now in a position to follow up our initial communication with a reinforced message - but before we did this, we approached the authorities.

And something strange happened. In the meantime, over the last few days, our supplier had disputed the validity of our test results. Then, after the international credentials of the laboratory were established, they had blocked and rejected our attempt to audit the site. They claimed that we had not specified a zero level of pathogenic E. coli in the product, and therefore they were not liable for the issue. My boss commented that we had not specified a zero level of plutonium cyanide in the product either; they still had a legal obligation to provide safe food. We went to regulatory authorities, confident in our scientific risk assessment. But the supplier was, shall we say, "well connected" and initially the authorities were sceptical about our decisions.

Fortunately, common sense prevailed. The recall was approved. The product withdrawn. The supplier disapproved. And no-one was hurt.

This was the end of phase one and end of the issue. Coda: Only a couple of months after this case, there was an article in Food Safety News. A hard cheese product made with raw milk had been responsible for an outbreak of food poisoning caused by E. coli O157:H7. Twenty-one people were sickened, one person had died. That could have been us.

Later, in a second phase, someone raised the question: "Why are we permitting own brand cheese made with unpasteurized milk?"

It is a good question. In many countries, notably the USA, raw milk cheese is not permitted. In Europe, vulnerable populations - such as pregnant women - are instructed to avoid such products. Why did we want to take such risks?

Here was my answer:

In quality and food safety, our job is to "Walk the Line" between maintaining regular availability of a wide range of food products, while keeping risks to a minimum. The only way to assure safety 100% at all times would be not to sell any food at all. Even the best food safety plans can never protect against all eventualities and could therefore ultimately be seen as practical compromises (which is why we need to be careful with statements such as "no compromise on food safety"). That can never be an excuse for negligence or poor management practices, or for a lack of vigilance and continuous improvement efforts. Still, the uncomfortable but unavoidable truth is that absolute guarantees of safety are not realistic.

In the case of raw milk cheese, there are powerful lobbies. One that sprang to my mind, as a Brit, was the passionate advocacy of Prince Charles, but even his enthusiasm for unpasteurized milk cheese pales in comparison to that of the great nation of France.

Removing raw milk cheese from the portfolio of our stores in an Eastern European country is one thing, but banning it from our stores in France? Ce n'est pas possible.

So, I created a working group, led by our French colleagues. Pasteurization, I said, is a well-known and globally accepted method to eliminate relevant pathogens from milk. How do you ensure that the raw milk cheese we sell is comparably safe?

The answer requires a much deeper dive into the value chain and includes the livestock health and sanitary status, the milking parlor hygiene, the storage and transport of the raw milk, and the cheese processing itself. It is more work, but the combination of well-managed hurdles can give an equivalent result to the CCP concept of pasteurization (72C for 15 s).

We formalized this French best practice into our internal Quality System.

Discussion and key learnings

This story illustrates several important points. Although the presence of E. coli is per se not the evidence of a health risk for consumers, it is an indication that there were hygiene problems in the production of cheese, and as such the conditions for ensuring safety have been compromised. This is all the more important since the cheese produced was made of raw milk and its safety relied on good hygienic practice. The rapid recall of products on the worst-case scenario assumption and on the precautionary principle was fully justified. In this case, it was even proven necessary. It spared the company from a serious food safety incident.

The question of cheese made from raw milk has been the subject of controversies and conflict between different countries and cultures. Although pasteurization of milk provides a safe method of production, experience has shown that it is possible to reach an equal degree of safety by using a combination of hurdles and applying good hygienic practice.

When managing a food safety crisis, the communication needs to be clear, decisive, and science-based. The priority concerns should be first, the safety of people then the regulatory compliance and last business continuity.

Further reading

- Food Safety News, 2013. Additional E. Coli O157:H7 Illness from Gort's Gouda Cheese Surfaces. https://www.foodsafetynews. com/2013/11/additional-e-coli-o157h7-illness-   linked-to-gorts-gouda-cheese-surfaces/, November 15, 2013.
- Motarjemi, Y., 2014. Hazard analysis and critical control point system (HACCP). In: Motarjemi, Y., Lelieveld, H. (Eds.), Food Safety Management: A Practical Guide for the Food Industry. Academic Press, Waltham MA, pp. 845-871.
- Reitsma, C.J., Henning, D.R., 1996. Survival of enterohemorrhagic Escherichia coli O157:H7 during the manufacture and curing of cheddar cheese. J. Food Protect. 59 (5), 460-464.

- Schlesser, J.E., Gerdes, R., Ravishankar, S., Madsen, K., Mowbray, J., Teo, A.Y., 2006. Survival of a five-strain cocktail of Escherichia coli O157:H7 during the 60-day aging period of cheddar cheese made from unpasteurized milk. J. Food Protect. 69 (5), 990-998.
- US Food and Drug Administration, 2016. Summary Report: Raw Milk Cheeses Aged 60 Days. Center for Food Safety and Applied Nutrition.

3.10 A process override

In an EU country, the company received consumer complaints about canned meat products, produced in-house in the same country. Cans were bulging. At that point there were two possibilities: (1) underprocessing or (2) leaking cans. Anyway, in both cases there was microbial contamination and growth. The company decided to issue a public recall immediately and subsequently informed the local authorities. Also, further production was halted and an investigation into the incident was initiated.

The local authorities were very critical of the recall, demanding to know what exactly was the nature of the microbial contamination, arguing that this situation was in all probability not a danger to public health and warning the company not to issue any public recalls on their own initiative ever again, but to inform them first and wait for instructions.

Later, the company understood that the reason the local authorities were contesting the recall was only because the news of the recall had already reached the central authorities in the capital city, who immediately contacted the local branch with questions they could not answer at the time.

Canned product was supposed to be sterilized in a steam retort, which was preconditioned by blowing steam through for 7 min. The investigation found that factory operators considered this process to be wasteful in terms of energy and too noisy. They managed to change the computer-controlled process in such a way that preconditioning now only lasted 2 min, which they deemed sufficient without any further validation. Subsequent heat mapping of the retort under these conditions showed a highly irregular heat distribution, leading to significant local underprocessing. No problems with can integrity were found.

Discussion and key learnings

1. Always and immediately recall canned products that are bulging. It may not be clear what the nature of the contamination is exactly, but danger to public health is a realistic possibility and there is no time to try and find out first.
2. Coordinate the recall with the local authorities and prevent a situation where local authorities are blindsided and unable to answer questions from their superiors.
3. Where food safety-related process parameters are computer controlled, make sure these settings cannot be changed/overridden by operators.
4. Explain the process to operators in advance, and when they raise concerns about energy use and noise (or any other aspect), explain again and address the concerns as much as possible (improved hearing protection) without jeopardizing food safety.

3.11 Powdered raw material

When running chocolate cookies through metal detectors at the end of a production line, a manufacturer found great numbers of small metal particles in their product. Tracing the problem to its origins, the cocoa powder, sourced from a supplier in Europe, was found to be heavily contaminated with these particles. Production was halted and a Quality Assurance (QA) team was dispatched to the supplier to investigate.

The supplier explained the process and the Hazard Analysis Critical Control Points (HACCP) system. Cocoa butter was separated from the cocoa cake (the dry matter) in a massive hydraulic press, using a fine-meshed metal filter mat. Being subjected to enormous pressures, the filter mat would typically start breaking down piece by piece and the metal particles would be mixed with the cocoa cake. Downstream transport of the cake would be via a system of successive magnets that would remove the metal particles. Magnets would be cleaned on a regular basis. The cleaning was recorded, but not the amount of metal removed. At fixed intervals, the filter mats would be replaced. By that time, they were usually well-worn. The system seemed to work as intended for a number of years, until one press mat did not break down piece by piece but all at once, catastrophically. Upon a regular daily visual inspection, the operators noticed, stopped the process, replaced the mat, cleaned the magnets, and started the process up again. The cocoa cake produced was shipped.

The joint investigation team concluded that the entire process was flawed for a number of reasons. There was an implicit acceptance of the mats having started to break down by the time they were being replaced, which always should have been considered as risky. There was also an assumption that the magnets would always be capable of eliminating any metal debris. This was never validated and, in all probability, should have been considered unrealistic from the start. The possibility of an earlier and more severe breakdown than normal was not considered, let alone a sudden catastrophic disintegration of the entire mat. Finally, and as a result of all this, there was no criterion by which the plant could conclude that the cocoa cake produced could be considered clean.

A new process was designed and implemented, where:

- Press mats would typically be replaced before they would start breaking down at intervals based on available historic information and ongoing monitoring.
- Capability tests would be carried out under controlled conditions to ascertain the magnet system's ability to eliminate all metal particles from cocoa cake under realistic conditions.
- Material recovered from the magnets to be inspected, weighed, and recorded. Action limits to be set for stopping the process and further investigation before starting up again. This way the magnets were used not only as a corrective measure but also as an ongoing check on the integrity of the mats.
- A "last magnet" to be installed that would have to remain clean at all times. If any metal particle would be found on this magnet, that would be seen as an indication that the material produced would be contaminated. That material would have to be carefully run over clean magnets again - if no metal was found at that stage, it could be shipped.

Discussion and key learnings

- A HACCP system must be designed to deal with a realistic hazard (in this case metal particles) in principle, but also under worst-case realistic conditions (if the whole mat breaks down suddenly, how much metal comes down the pipe? Can our magnets deal with that?).

- HACCP systems require quantitative action limits - in this case, there were none.
- Setting replacement intervals for safety-critical parts of equipment at the moment the hazard typically already manifests itself is asking for trouble. This supplier needed to change over to data-based preventive maintenance.
- Operators who find an abnormal situation (press mat suddenly disintegrated) with potential food safety consequences must alert QA - and must have been instructed to do so - before continuing.

3.12 Suspicious meatballs?

This story is from a reputable catering firm in Istanbul, Turkey, which provides foodservice to various clients/customers, including private enterprises, government agencies, schools, hospitals, and, in this case, a top media company.

One of the regular catering items is a meatball, a popular Turkish food, which comes in various forms. Generally, ground beef and mutton, multiple spices, bread, minced onion and garlic, parsley, and egg are the ingredients used in the recipes. These recipes may often be specified in the catering contract with a customer, which then becomes legally binding. At the same time, however, meatballs may often be susceptible to adulteration. The most common trick to reduce the cost is by using soy mince as a filler, against contractual specifications. It counts as adulteration, but it cannot be detected sensorially. One day, the director of the catering firm in question applied to our university's food safety laboratory with some meatball samples, as delivered to the aforementioned media company and said that personnel from that customer had complained about the quality of the meatball. They claimed that it was not produced from meat, but only included soy mince. Also, soy being inherently genetically modified, this then would lead to an accusation of food fraud and adulteration and a violation of the foodservice contract terms. Naturally, we asked how the claimant knew. The foodservice company's director gave us the test obtained from a food quality control laboratory by the claimant. The test report said that the meatball contained genetically modified soy mince. However, the Director of catering claimed that he never used soy mince in making meatballs and produced his meatballs wholly from beef mince.

We investigated the claim. Initial DNA and polymerase chain reaction (PCR) screening confirmed that the meatball samples indeed consisted of beef mince. But there was more in the recipe, it included various spices, salt, oil, and some dried and ground bread for binding the meatball. It was the ground bread that caught our attention. The Turkish Food Codex allows the use of soy protein in bakery products, including bread, to increase its nutritional status. And so, we did a PCR test to screen the soy sauce as used in the bread. It turned out positive for genetically modified (GM) soy, not really surprising as almost 85% of all soy worldwide is GM.

We prepared a test report for the catering operator to share with their customer, explaining all relevant details.

Discussion and key learnings

This case illustrates the different perspectives of customers and caterers. The customer wanted an assurance of safe food, in accordance with the specification and without adulteration, which they felt also included any trace of genetically modified organisms (GMOs). In the accusation, the customer did not follow due process, did not present much verifiable evidence, and simply assumed that soy mince had been used as a filler, the most common trick to reduce the cost, against the specifications in the contract.

In our investigation, the accusation against the caterer proved mostly unfounded - meatballs were made from beef and not from soy mince. Still, soy was being used, albeit in the context of the ground bread and according to applicable regulations. As the large majority of soy globally is GM, our findings in that regard were not surprising. So, there was a bit of truth in the allegations after all, but no fraud, no adulteration, and nothing illegal. The lab test on which the claim of fraud was supposed to be based should never have formulated in a way that seemed to support a claim that the meatballs actually mostly consisted of soy mince.

Additionally:

Trust is good but, for due diligence purposes, it is a good practice to check:

- Customers need to check and verify that their supplier is conforming to requirements.
- Providers need to also validate and verify to ensure their food safety systems and always be prepared to respond to queries and challenges.
- Complaints of any kind need to be taken seriously and when a company's products and practices are put in question, the company will have to be well prepared to respond quickly.
- Now, probably more than in the past, rumors may spread quickly and there will always be people who simply believe what they may hear and read, also without any substantial evidence.
- As a customer, or laboratory, it is important not to draw hasty conclusions in the interpretation of the results and have an open dialogue with the supplier.
- In working with outside labs, you need to know exactly what you are asking for and how to interpret results.
- QA people will need to anticipate on complaints, accusations, and rumors; they need to guard against any unauthorized deviations of agreed recipes and make sure the integrity and authenticity of the products is documented on an ongoing basis. And, probably like no other function, QA knows that the devil is in the details.

3.13 The role of laboratory surveillance in the detection of outbreaks

Listeria monocytogenes is a bacterium that causes a rare but severe disease in susceptible individuals - listeriosis. It is one of the most feared foodborne pathogens: the most frequent cause of death from contaminated food in Europe and one of the deadliest of all bacteria. In addition to suffering, functional disability, and death, L. monocytogenes and listeriosis have a huge economic and environmental impact. Not only the health systems but also the food industry is severely affected. Food recalls frequently result in the destruction of large amounts of foods, brand damage, lost sales, and litigation costs, among others.

In Portugal, notification of cases of listeriosis is mandatory only since April 2014, so no official published data have been available until 2016 (EFSA, 2016). In the absence of a nationally implemented listeriosis surveillance system, in 2003, a voluntary collaboration was established between the main hospitals in Portugal (covering about 90% of the population) and the Center for Biotechnology and Fine Chemistry (CBQF) - the research center of Escola Superior de Biotecnologia (CBQF) - with the aim of collecting data on listeriosis in the country and characterizing clinical isolates of L. monocytogenes, both phenotypically and genetically. Although not "official," the first data on the incidence of listeriosis in Portugal, based on retrospective information provided by the hospitals, were published in 2006 (Almeida et al., 2006) - "Listeriosis in Portugal: an existing but under-reported infection." In 2010, another publication reported an increase in the prevalence of the infection between 2003 and 2007 (Magalhaes et al., 2014).

Between January and July 2010, we were suddenly confronted with an exceptional increase in the number of listeriosis cases, most of these in the Lisbon and Vale do Tejo region (LVTR). Very worrying was the fact that these cases were probably interrelated - the isolates recovered from patients revealed a similar restriction profile when typed by pulsed-field gel electrophoresis (PFGE). We had no doubt that there was an ongoing outbreak, with people dying. At that stage, we alerted the Directorate-General of Health (DGS) who officially declared an outbreak.

What a pressure, mainly by journalists who reported: "There are already more than 20 cases and 13 deaths since the beginning of the year."

An investigation was started. Epidemiological questionnaires were administered to the patients or their families. "Queijo fresco," cured cheese, ice cream, ham, and "alheira" (a traditional Portuguese fermented sausage) were identified as possible sources of transmission. Based on these data, concerning the suspected foods, type of establishments where the products were bought, and geographical location of the cases, the Portuguese Food Safety Authority (ASAE) collected food and environmental samples for microbiological analysis. Positive samples were found but no match between food and clinical isolates. On October 29, 2010, during a working meeting to discuss the outbreak investigation with DGS, an excited student came in: we did it! The outbreak strain was detected "queijo fresco" samples collected in two markets in LVTR and produced by two different companies. We were almost there. The next step was the collection of samples in these companies, before being delivered to the market (November 2010eMarch 2011). Positive samples were only detected in samples of one of the companies and L. monocytogenes isolates from cheeses shared the same pulsotype as the clinical isolates. Cheeses produced by this company were considered the probable source of the outbreak. Cross-contamination of cheeses from the other company may have occurred in the market as cheeses produced by both companies were sold in the two local markets. After this, ASAE proceeded to recall these products, more samples were analyzed (March 2011), and cheeses made with cow and goat milk tested positive for L. monocytogenes (outbreak pulsotype). At this stage the factory agreed to a voluntary suspension and after disinfection more cheese and environmental samples were collected. As no positive samples were detected, product was delivered again to the market. Samples were then collected by ASAE on a monthly basis but no more positives were detected.

Discussion and key learnings

Although this was the first detected and confirmed outbreak of listeriosis recorded in Portugal, being one of the most serious worldwide (fatality rate 36.7%), evidence was found that other outbreaks, involving a smaller number of cases, may have occurred without being detected and reported (Magalhaes et al., 2015).

The magnitude of this outbreak and the long period from its detection to its termination highlight the importance of having an effective listeriosis surveillance system and investigation procedures in place for early detection and resolution of outbreaks. Advances in our capacity to match food with outbreak strains by PFGE and more recently by whole genome sequencing are enabling the detection of outbreaks earlier than what was previously possible and even to detect outbreaks that would have gone unnoticed in the past.

In this case the investigation was limited to epidemiological aspects and recall of incriminated products. However, in any incident it is important to make a root cause analysis and find out the reason for contamination of products.

References

- Almeida, G.N., Gibbs, P.A., Hogg, T.A., Teixeira, P., 2006. Listeriosis in Portugal: an existing but under reported infection. BMC Infect. Dis. 6, 153. https://doi.org/10.1186/1471-2334- 6-153.
- EFSA (European Food Safety Authority) and ECDC (European Centre for Disease Prevention and Control), 2016. The European Union summary report on trends and sources of zoonoses, zoonotic agents and food-borne outbreaks in 2015. EFSA J. 14 (12). https://doi.org/ 10.2903/j.efsa.2016.4634, 4634, 231 pp.
- Magalhaes, R., Ferreira, V., Santos, I., Almeida, G., Teixeira, P., Research Team, 2014. Genetic and phenotypic characterization of Listeria monocytogenes from human clinical cases that occurred in Portugal between 2008 and 2012. Foodborne Pathogen. Dis. 11 (11), 907-916. https://doi.org/10.1089/fpd.2014.1806.
- Magalhaes, R., Almeida, G., Ferreira, V., Santos, I., Silva, J., Mendes, M.M., Pita, J., Mariano, G., Mancio, I., Sousa, M.M., Farber, J., Pagotto, F., Teixeira, P., 2015. Cheese-related listeriosis outbreak, Portugal, March 2009 to February 2012. Euro Surveill. 20 (17). https://doi.org/10.2807/1560-7917.ES2015.20.17.21104.

3.14 One way trip: pathogen environmental monitoring program

By training and professional experience, my company had designated me as a "Food Safety-Microbiology Subject Matter Expert" and I therefore was the "right person" for a difficult situation. I was called in to the office of the Vice President and was told that I have a "one-way trip." The multinational company was a market confectionery leader and had recently acquired a regional company. Unfortunately, the regional company had a facility in South America that had several successive recalls with Salmonella in their chocolate products. My assignment was to assess the situation and determine if things could quickly be resolved. The "One Way Trip" was to impress on me the gravity of the situation.

Before taking a red-eye flight, I made several calls to the facility and reviewed in detail the list of sensitive ingredients (SI), which may be described as ingredients that are likely to have been associated with pathogens based on origin, historical, epidemiological data, and where the primary microbiological hazard control is managed by the supplier (and with no pathogen inactivation by the customer or in end use by consumers). Of the SI list, I was particularly interested in sesame seeds that were regionally produced and used in the chocolate products. The regional Food Safety and Supplier Quality Assurance teams assured me that the sesame seed processing has been validated to exceed five logs pathogen inactivation. To their frustration, they had not been able to pinpoint the source of the Salmonella that showed up on a regular basis in the Pathogen Environmental Monitoring (PEM) Program. A visit to the sesame seed supplier confirmed that there was the roasting as an effective kill step. However, the supplier also produced raw sesame seeds and both products used post roaster shared equipment with dry cleaning for packaging operation.

The facility was a very old converted multiple story brick building with wood floors, and it had seen better days. Parts of the roof were damaged and prone to leaks.

A maintenance crew had installed temporary ceiling leak diverters (that became permanent) and makeshift rain gutters that diverted water through the processing halls. The regional Food Safety Team considered that Salmonella can be associated with birds and would like to expand the PEM program to include the roof.

Under the circumstances, however, hygienic conditions could not be restored and moving production to a brand-new facility was the only effective solution.

Discussion and key learnings

Salmonella had ingress into the facility's infrastructure and the facility could not be saved. There are cases where Salmonella has been demonstrated to be able to survive for multiple years in a low moisture environment.

There were too many potential vectors into the facility from leaking roofs, inappropriate use of material and structures (i.e., wood floors, internal rain gutters), as well as questionable SI. The facility relied heavily on PEM as the primary control measure when in fact PEM is only a verification of the Pathogen Control Program. The Grocery Manufacture of America provides guidance for control of Salmonella in low moisture foods, which readily applies to this situation:

1. Prevent ingress or spread of Salmonella in the processing facility (facility floors, walls, roof, etc.)
2. Enhance the stringency of hygiene practices and controls in the Primary Salmonella Control Area (the entire facility proceeding area would be considered a primary control area as there are no pathogen kill step or separate distinct zoning)
3. Apply hygienic design principles to building and equipment design (equipment should be accessible for inspection and cleaning)
4. Prevent or minimize growth of Salmonella within the facility (minimize the use of water in cleaning-sanitization)
5. Establish a raw materials/ingredients control program (i.e., Supplier Quality Assurance Program, validated kill step, and Pathogen Certificate of Analysis [CoA] available before use)
6. Validate control measures to inactivate Salmonella (for SI)
7. Establish procedures for verification of Salmonella controls and corrective actions (PEM Program)
8. Sometimes, despite the costs, effectively controlling a risk requires drastic measures such as changing the design of a product or even building an entirely new facility, as demonstrated in this story.

Further reading

- Grocery Manufacturer Association (GMA), 2009. Control of Salmonella in Low Moisture Foods. http://graphics8.nytimes.com/packages/pdf/business/20090515_moss_ingredients/SalmonellaControlGuidance.pdf
- WHO, 2008. Foodborne Disease Outbreaks – Guideline for Investigation and Control. https:// www.who.int/foodsafety/publications/foodborne_disease/outbreak_guidelines.pdf.

3.15 Fish soup intoxication: where is the investigation?

Once upon a time, when 10 countries were queuing up to become member states of the European Union, much had to be done, including the harmonization of food legislation, part of the so-called *acquis communautaire*.

Together with a number of other experts, I was sent to a candidate country, one of those having most troubles with food safety, even basic hygiene.

At that time, I was a young expert, enthusiastic, and full of willingness to help and share my knowledge, both in terms of food safety and of EU food law. The mission was organized in the framework of a project called PHARE.

As a token of appreciation, we were one evening invited to a very good and widely known local restaurant in the capital, a fish restaurant. I came from a landlocked country where the fish consumption is very low, so I was happy to spend the night in great company and treated with good fish dishes. When the waiter wanted to take my order, I asked for any kind of fish. For most fishes, I didn't know their names, not even in my mother tongue. In brief, I asked for a very hot fish soup and a very well-cooked fried or grilled fish, whatever the type was. As an expert in food safety, knowing risks with potentially contaminated food during travel, I wanted to act responsibly and chose a hot and well-done food which presents the lowest microbial risks. However, still, this precautionary measure was not enough and did not help, as many toxins or hazards of chemical nature are heat resistant.

The dinner was nice. The colleagues from the host country were very kind, but next morning when we were awaited by a van to be taken to the sites for the day's meetings and site visits, I felt quite sick. I am not particularly sensitive, and I consider myself to have a very high tolerance for pain, but this time I felt awful. I had nausea, headache, and more. I felt like vomiting any minute and above all my hands were shaking uncontrollably. It was a horrifying experience. I was grateful to have my colleagues from my home country with me. I had to get out of the van even before getting in and I do not remember anything of the hours which followed. I am told that I was walked back to my hotel room and I missed that day.

The next morning, I queried the hosts, who had taken the same order in the restaurant. He was a veterinarian, a big man, possibly over 100 kg. He mentioned that we had exactly the same fish soup and fish meal and started to joke about it. I wanted to know if he had any health issues after having consumed the meal. He mentioned that he had a little bit of stomach ache, but nothing serious.

Unfortunately, more preoccupied to get on with our duties, we did not report the case and there was no investigation as to the cause of the case.

Discussion and key learnings

- Although one cannot fully prevent adverse events, during travels, as a precautionary measure, it is important to choose foods which present the minimum risks.
- In hindsight, I recognize that although we were experts on the subject of food safety, at the time we behaved exactly as most consumers. That is, as soon as we got well, we went on with our work without reporting the case. Subsequently, there was no investigation and improvement of the hygiene

in the restaurant. This general situation makes that there is a high degree of underreporting of foodborne illnesses.

- In the absence of an investigation, it is not known what kind of illness we suffered, what was the agent of the intoxication, which kind of fish was the culprit, if the intoxication was of microbial or chemical origin, such as histamine, and what was the level of the agent.
- Different factors can explain the difference in the clinical manifestation of the illness. Even if we ordered the same food, did we actually get the same? Was there the same level of contamination? Were there interfering factors such as an underlying medical condition or was there a medication that heightened the impact of intoxication? Who else got ill?
- Assuming that we, both patients, ate the same amount, was it the difference in bodyweight that made us react differently? That is the dose-per-kilogram response principle, commonly used in toxicology.
- In an outbreak, members of a cohort may react differently. Each incidents merits a thorough investigation to not only stop the process of intoxication but also to learn about the risk profile of foodborne diseases.

Chapter Four

Hazard and risk assessment

4.1 Process sampling lessons learned

I began my industrial statistics career with a fruit and vegetable packing company. Fresh out of graduate school, I was more than a little nervous about inspiring new colleagues to make data-driven decisions through the use of statistically designed experiments and to improve manufacturing processes by using methods associated with statistical process control.

A first major opportunity came my way when Leo darkened my door. Introducing himself as an industrial engineer, he explained that he was working on a project to assess the effectiveness of the lye peeler to aid in removing the skins but not pulp of tomatoes for further processing. Leo went on to describe the peeling process. Then we ventured into the nearby cannery to watch it in operation.

To my naïve eyes, it seemed designed to prohibit sampling. Tomatoes rushed through a flume at breakneck speed into a tangle of slicers, dicers, cookers, and who-knows-what-ers before the canning, palletizing, and warehousing operations. I left with more questions than answers, but we returned to my office to discuss sampling.

I must admit to being overwhelmed by what I perceived as the process complexity and the seeming difficulty of obtaining fair, unbiased pre- and post- processing samples. May I have some time to consider, and may we meet again next day, I asked Leo.

A sleepless night followed. My young bride wondered why I was so worried and if there might be lye in our diced tomatoes. With the dawn, I had a scheme which I believed would prove effective at providing Leo with a workable solution and give him the answers he needed.

We met, I presented my recommended plan, and then he informed me of what he had intended to do all along, no matter what I had suggested. I turned beet- or tomato-red; I was furious at being led along in this manner, and I did something I should not have done. I told Leo I could not help him and that I must move on to other work. Good luck.

Later that week, Leo went to the cannery, stuck 20 differently colored pins into each of 20 tomatoes, weighed each, and sent them through the lye peeler.

He recovered 18.

Discussion and key learnings

Leo had made up his mind in advance and had no intention to listen to the advice he requested. As a result, two pins may have gone out to consumers. This is a dangerous situation, to say the least. Industrial statisticians are there to help companies make informed decisions, based on actual data that are collected in the course of valid experiments. If your company has a statistician, ask the statistician for advice if you plan an experiment - not just as a formality. If your company does not have a statistician, hire a consultant, especially in pivotal situations.

- Experiments on a product that is meant to be sold must be planned and carried out with the utmost care. Under no circumstances should there be any potential risk to consumers as a result of the experiment.
- Foreign bodies resulting from experiments or otherwise are always a realistic possibility in production. Processing lines must include protections against foreign bodies.

Further reading

- Box, G.E.P., Hunter, J.S., Hunter, W.G., 2005. Statistics for Experimenters. John Wiley and Sons, New York.
- Hoerl, R., Snee, R., 2020. Statistical Thinking, third ed. Wiley, Hoboken, NJ.
- Montgomery, D.C., 2013a. Design and Analysis of Experiments, eighth ed. John Wiley and Sons, New York.
- Montgomery, D.C., 2013b. Introduction to Statistical Quality Control, seventh ed. John Wiley and Sons, Hoboken, NJ.
- Snee, R.D., Hare, L.B., Trout, J.R. (Eds.), 1985. Experiments in Industry. American Society for Quality, Milwaukee, WI.

4.2 Binomial coffee milk cups

In an EU country, a coffee-producing company decided to start producing coffee milk cups, sterilized in a retort. The production was planned in a facility that had no previous experience with retorted cups, and neither had the company, although high-level canning expertise was available.

Apart from the proper thermal processing conditions, the microbiological stability (commercial sterility) of this kind of product will depend on the structural integrity of the cups. Are they and will they remain hermetically sealed during retorting and later under normal transport and storage conditions? The Quality Assurance and Food Safety (QA/FS) department felt that this needed to be established before the product would be launched. To this end, they needed to answer two questions: (1) what would be an appropriate failure level? and (2) how to test for that? Production staff felt that a proper installation of the filling and cup sealing equipment by an experienced supplier should be sufficient, but QA/FS insisted that their questions be properly answered.

A quantitative target for the structural integrity failure rate of cans or cups proved hard to find. At the time, only Canadian legislation mentioned - for cans - an allowable failure rate of 1 in 10,000, stating this was a statistical approximation. In the absence of other applicable standards, this was accepted as the target. The second question was how to test for that. Production proposed to produce 10,000 cups, submerge them in a water bath, and expose them to an as-yet unspecified mild underpressure to find leakers. QA/FS had in the meantime spoken to colleagues in the industry who informed them that they did not work with an a priori overall failure rate (1 in 10,000 or otherwise), but used a two-step process: for each production batch a number of cups would be tested in a water bath with mild underpressure (no failures allowed) and subsequently with more severe underpressure (fixed maximum number of failures allowed). This was seen as a practical approach for ongoing production, but not for the initial approval of the targeted 1 in 10,000 or better process capability. Applying the milder level of underpressure, QA/FS proposed to run a test that would provide a 95% certainty that the process would perform at the targeted failure level. According to the binomial distribution table (reference below), 30,000 (actually 29,956) samples would have to be tested, with no failures found, to reach the 95% confidence level. Production balked.

A huge debate ensued, around the target (why would Canadian legislation apply to Europe?), around the level of underpressure (why would we have to follow the technical practices of competitors?), around the need for acceptance testing of the first production (why can't we just use the much simpler acceptance procedure of the equipment supplier? Or use the technical practices of competitors?), and most of all around the conclusions from the binomial table (entirely theoretical, impractical, and a huge waste).

The fact that QA/FS was represented on the board of the company, independent from production, ultimately made a compromise possible. There would be a test with 30,000 cups being produced and tested, with two failures allowed at most if a subsequent root cause investigation would lead to an identifiable and repairable cause. And so it went - and with a minor adjustment of the installation, proper production could begin.

Discussion and key learnings

- QA/FS needs to have board-level representation, independent from production, in order to make sure

disputes can get elevated and decided at the appropriate senior level, if necessary.
- Acceptance testing requirements for new products or processes need to be agreed upon at an early stage.
- Criteria need to be quantitative and properly explained to stakeholders.
- QA/FS needs to have a professional network, enabling them to consult colleagues in the industry.

Further reading

- Diep, B., Moulin, J., Bastic-Schmid, V., Putallaz, T., Gimonet, J., Deban Valles, A., Klijn, A., September, 2019. Validation protocol for commercial sterility testing methods. Food Contr. 103, 1-8.
- Johnson, N.L., Kemp, A.W., Kotz, S., September, 2005. Univariate Discrete Distributions, third ed. Wiley.

4.3 May contain peanut

A European company made a chocolate product that was labeled as "may contain peanuts," because peanuts were used in the same facility (facility "A") and cross-contact could not be entirely prevented. The situation was stable for years, with the product being sold across a number of countries, without any allergen- related complaints.

Then, the product was moved to another existing production site (facility "B") where it was also produced under "may contain" conditions and distributed across Europe as before. Within days, the company received several complaints of serious allergic reactions, mostly from long-time consumers who knew themselves to be allergic to peanuts. Despite the fact the product was labeled as "may contain peanuts" and the consumers who complained were clearly aware of the warnings, the company decided that the situation was serious enough to warrant a public recall.

In a subsequent investigation, it was found that products made at facility B could contain far higher levels of peanut than before. The B site produced mostly nut- containing products and the product in question was always produced on a line that had run a nut-containing variety immediately before. Chocolate production lines are typically not wet-cleaned, but the remnants of the "old" product are pushed out by the new and so the first chocolate bars of a new production run were always mixed with relatively high levels of the previous - nut-containing - product.

Interviews with the consumers who complained revealed that they tested themselves against what was available on the market. They would carefully try a "may contain" product, and if a tiny bit did not seem to affect them, they would go on and eat it. Assuming the product would always be the same, they would then simply start eating a subsequent purchase, without testing a small bite first. When the product produced at plant B arrived on the shelves, they were suddenly confronted with a significantly higher nut level than what they had expected and immediately suffered severe reactions.

Having completed the recall, the company had to decide under what conditions the product could be reintroduced, as they did not want to move production back to facility A. In the absence of clear guidance as to what "may contain" would actually mean in terms of levels of allergens in a product, an ad hoc target had to be set. Comparisons with the old product from facility A, a literature study, and discussions with toxicologists led to a target level of 25 ppm being decided upon. Under the existing production regime at site B that was clearly unrealistic, two routes were considered:

1. At the changeover from nut-containing to nut-free products to reject the first product flow until all nuts were washed out and levels consistently below 25 ppm were reached. This was found to be too expensive and wasteful, with high amounts of product being rejected.
2. A wet cleaning of the line before the nut-free production would start. Attempts proved to be too time-intensive and were deemed to be risky from a microbiological perspective, even under the most controlled conditions.

Ultimately, it was decided to move production to another nut-free facility, which would then also allow the removal of the "may contain" labeling entirely.

Discussion and key learnings

- Any change in production should result in a re-evaluation of the safety of the products, the presence of possible allergens and their amounts, including anticipation of consumer behavior and response, and the need to change the safety information on the packaging.
- Allergic consumers will try "may contain" products and test themselves. If they don't experience any symptoms, they may be less cautious with a subsequent purchase. Changing production practices and de facto allergen levels may then pose a risk.
- Setting realistic quantitative limits for "may contain" is exceedingly difficult, also in the light of the above. A probabilistic risk assessment may be the best way to go about this (see reference).
- Especially in a confectionery environment, effective cleaning/separation regimes may not be feasible. Concentrating production in all- or no-allergen facilities appears to be the safest route.

Further reading

Remington, B.C., Baumert, J.L., Marx, D.B., Taylor, S.L., December, 2013. Quantitative risk assessment of foods containing peanut advisory labelling. Food Chem. Toxicol. 62, 179-187.

4.4 Why is the food not warm enough?

The year was 2007 when Romania just entered the European Union (EU) and recently harmonized its food safety legislation with the EU aquis. At the food safety symposium, experienced guests and renowned keynote speakers in food safety, from Europe and the United States, were invited. Numerous specialists took part in the debates. To demonstrate commitment to the food safety values and to provide meals at the meeting, the enthusiastic organizers decided to select a local catering company that implemented the Hazard Analysis Critical Control Point (HACCP) principles and had a food safety certification and bragged about it to all participants.

At the meeting, the weather was nice and warm, the atmosphere was friendly, and the presentations were very stimulating. The symposium was a real success given the attending stakeholders and the interesting discussions, while food was tasty, nutritionally balanced with a nice selection of desserts, fruits, and vegetables, next to the main courses, delivered on time and attractively presented by the caterer.

However, at some point, the organizers had to respond to a very simple question that popped up from one US keynote speakers at the Symposium. The sharp question was: "Why the warm food is not warm enough and the deserts and salads are not cold enough"?

Discussion and key learnings

Obviously, the inability of caterers to ensure that food is outside the temperature danger zone (5-57.5°C) throughout the entire conference duration demonstrated that, although there was a declared commitment to food safety values, not all the food safety measures were well understood and implemented.

To demonstrate a functional HACCP system in food catering, it is not enough to have a well paper-documented food safety system, but it needs to control hazards, obstinately follow the food safety principles, and give priority to basic rules of hygiene from raw materials purchase to food delivery. Thus, in this case, potentially hazardous food should not linger in the temperature danger zone more than 2 h, because it could allow pathogens' growth.

Disregarding simple food safety rules can sometimes be easily spotted by specialists by the naked eye and these observations made not only the organizers of the event feel embarrassed, but also it could have compromised the entire organizational effort and, in the worst-case scenario, produced an outbreak.

In this case, "all's well that ends well" and no illnesses were reported, but the lesson learnt was powerful and became a classic case study among the food safety practitioners and students in Romania.

4.5 Meat with salmonella or without salmonella?

It was in the 1990s and I was working in a public health institute. Salmonella infections were on the rise in most industrialized countries. Poultry meat was one of the identified vectors. Public health authorities were intensifying the education of professional and domestic food handlers.

One day, with my mother, I went into a shop, a butcher's shop, where they sold meat and other products such as delicatessen. In the shop, there was the butcher, a man in his fifties, and then his assistant, a young woman. She was cleaning the chickens and removing the guts. We asked for about 200 g of slices of ham. The lady stopped her work and went to the other part of the shop, where the charcuterie was on display, to cut us the ham that we had asked for.

Immediately, my mother and I thought of the same thing. We got nervous about what she was doing. Too careful not to offend her, I was thinking about how to express our concern, that my mother, more assertive, nudged me and whispered in my ear: Say something!

So, carefully and politely, I said: Madam, you know that raw chicken can be dangerous. Don't you?

She looked at me with a bewildered expression and said: So what?

I continued: Well, chicken can be contaminated with salmonella and there is a risk of cross- contamination from serving us ham without washing your hands.

She did not respond and quietly went on to wash her hands and serve us. In the meantime, annoyed, the butcher intervened in the discussion. He had not fully realized the situation. He said angry: The chicken will be cooked, Ma'am! To this I replied: Yes, but I'm not buying chicken but cold ham that won't be cooked!

His attitude made me to further justify my intervention: I explained that I was working in the field of public health and that this was a public health measure that we recommend to all consumers.

On hearing the term public health, he started to mock the public health institutions.

As we were leaving the shop, a man came in and asked to buy some meat. In a derisive tone, the butcher asked him: Do you want meat with salmonella or without salmonella?

Discussions and key learnings

When I remember this story, it reminds me of another event when I was looking for a job. I was interviewed by the director of the research center of a supermarket chain. During the interview, the director of the center told me that in general, he did not like to recruit women for such jobs. He was referring to a manager position in a meat section. However, he said that with time he has realized that when a man says something to the workers, they say "yes," but as soon as the manager has left, workers continue with their old wrong practice. He now thinks that it is not as much a question of gender but of the way things are communicated.

This experience raises many questions. Firstly, the question of training and education of food handlers to persuade them of the need for food hygiene measures and also of consumers so that these are also attentive to hygienic measures and ask for it.

It is also about the perception of women versus men. Would the butcher have reacted in the same way if a man had raised the issue?

In this story, the butcher was an older man; he had always acted this way, and changing his behavior, especially in an area related to hygiene, can be seen as offensive and hurt his professional pride.

Education of food safety and hygiene must start in early childhood and education of school children is the most effective way.

4.6 It never rains in Southern California

One year, some time ago, there was a bumper crop of tomatoes in Southern California. The Chief Executive Officer (CEO) of a food packing company was eager to pack all the tomatoes possible even though storage facilities were inadequate to accommodate the estimated volume. Processing, canning, and packing proceeded at breakneck speed, and when the warehouse was filled to overflowing, the decision was made to stack pallets of product outdoors. Chances of rain in that region at that time of year were slim and none.

After the rain, crews were brought in to disassemble pallets, remove soggy corrugate and drenched paper labels, and then to towel dry and eliminate any rust from the cans in preparation for new labeling. Meanwhile, a hastily constructed temporary structure was appended to the existing warehouse. While not up to fire code for want of an overhead sprinkler system, it was filled with newly restored tomato products despite recommendations to the contrary by quality professionals boldly issuing career-limiting advice to the contrary.

During the deluge immediately following, the temporary warehouse collapsed, taking with it part of the original warehouse together with large portions of its intact overhead sprinkler system. Water from that system spilled over previously packed pallets of products. Promised profits perished.

It never rains in Southern California. But it did.

Discussion and key learnings

This is a classic example of mistaking a general rule (it rarely rains in Southern California) for a law of nature (rain does not fall in Southern California). In the subsequent panic, all rules, regulations, and professional advice were broken and ignored, and the whole thing ended in disaster.

Lessons:

- Do not think you can predict the weather.
- The rules are there for a reason - break them at your peril.
- Effective leadership does not panic. It builds an environment where specialist opinions - even when they are in the minority at the time - and words of caution are welcome.

4.7 Risk assessment of the vegetable oils and fats supply chains

In 1999, we found that a shipload of unrefined palm oil for my company was contaminated with diesel oil. This appeared to be an adulteration, which at that time appeared to be current practice in some parts of the world. We felt that a reliance on detection of contaminations at the port of arrival was not the way forward and we started an active risk assessment program of our most important sourcing areas of vegetable oils and fats in southeast Asia (palm and coconut oil), Brazil and the United States (soybean oil), South Africa and France (sunflower oil), and Germany (rapeseed oil).

These assessments were supported by contaminant analyses of oils and fats arriving at port and our refineries in South Africa and Germany.

Customer visits to vegetable oil producing companies and regions were not as common in these days as they are now (these days often replaced by external audits/certification) and we found that most of the visited companies were cooperative and interested in our recommendations for improvement, but one of the companies we visited had a low standard of housekeeping. Mineral oil residues leaking from waste drums could easily mix with crude palm oil during unloading of the road tankers and the management was not interested in our recommendations for improvement because the company mainly exported to China and India (and they had never received customer visits from those countries at that time) and hardly to Europe.

In another case, a grower of sunflower seeds was mainly concerned about Datura plants between the sunflowers, because the poisonous Datura seeds would be a feed safety hazard in the sunflower meal. We were more interested in the levels of pesticides, but we also suspected contamination with polycyclic aromatic hydrocarbons (PAHs) from the drying of the seeds using exhaust gasses of a diesel burner. However, Datura and PAH levels were at that time not in the contract and therefore not analyzed.

A similar situation was found with coconut. After harvesting, the coconuts were peeled, halved, and dried on a bamboo grid above the burning husks. Insufficient or too late drying of the halved coconuts led to high levels of aflatoxin in the copra and in the meal after oil extraction. The drying process over an open fire of relative wet burning husk resulted in high levels of PAHs in the copra and in the oil after extraction. The aflatoxin level in the meal was seen as a critical control point in the oil extraction plant, but the PAH level in the oil could not be analyzed locally and was therefore not considered to be a contaminant of concern.

Discussion and key learnings

- The situations described earlier are only some 15 years ago, but they illustrate some key learnings that have led to major improvements since then:
- A smaller customer's demands for food safety improvements may not be heard if they are not supported by (much) larger customers - so don't waste your time with such a supplier (but you need to go there to see and understand the situation yourself)
- A visit may also show that your original specification is incomplete, there may be realistic hazards (Datura, PAHs) that need to be included immediately in an updated spec.
- Drying over open fires (from diesel oil, or rubber tires) will cause high levels of contamination (PAHs) and

is unacceptable, but again you need to go and see the practices with your own eyes.

- The fact that a contaminant cannot be analyzed locally does not mean that it is no longer a concern.
- Building a good relationship with the partners in the supply chain is essential for these assessments. It was not the objective to approve or reject suppliers but to get a good insight in their way of working and the materials they were using. In return, many of the companies in the supply chains were very interested in our recommendations for improvement.
- The combination of supply chain visits and raw material analyses appeared to be a costly but effective way to assess the risk of contaminants presence in the raw materials. This led to the establishment of a risk matrix with a focused analytical program.
- There are large differences in cultural backgrounds in the various supply chains.

Knowledge of the culture, religion, and habits should be obtained before the execution of the assessment.

Further reading

van Duijn, G., 2014. Oils and Fats. In: Encyclopedia of Food Safety, vol. 3, pp. 315-323.

4.8 Variation, process understanding, and profitability

A society for quality professionals had invited me to present a 2-h overview of statistical process control. Just prior to my going into the meeting hall, a man greeted me and told me that he could not attend my session but that he had attended it the previous year. He went on to say that he had gotten a great deal of useful information out of it, but he had one question.

"Why don't your people do what you say they should do," he asked. I considered his question and was tempted to respond by telling him that I had a wife, three kids, two dogs, and a cat. None of them does what I tell them to do, so why should I expect anything different at work? Instead, I asked him if he could be more specific.

He told me that he was in charge of his company's X-ray division which used our gelatin as a substrate and that he was prepared to spend over $1.5 million to retool his process so he could switch over to another vendor. It seems our gelatin had metal filings in it, and physicians were alarmed that their patients may have taken a bullet when false signals lit up on their screens. They were seeking alternate sources for their X-ray plates.

That was on a Friday. The following Monday, I phoned my friend George who was the CEO of the responsible subsidiary. I explained how I had encountered the hostile customer and learned of his threat. "That's a third of our business," exclaimed George. "What the heck are you doing giving short courses, anyway?"

George apologized immediately. He knew better than to shoot the messenger. He expressed profound concern over the threat to that business. Certainly, it spilled over to his food grade gelatin business, as well. "How soon can you get out to the plant and provide some help," he asked.

Two weeks later, I visited the plant. In the meantime, the plant manager had been alerted and, at my suggestion, had divided his workforce into teams associated with each of the manufacturing process unit operations. The goal was to create greater product consistency - less batch-to-batch variation - and to gain greater control over the process. Lacking was an in-depth understanding of all process unit operations.

My initial role was to meet with each of the unit operation teams to help them get started. The first team worked at the very beginning of the process and consisted of a mix of new and experienced operators, some of whom learned the process operation via on-the-job training. We started by discussing the process flow, and I showed examples of process flow diagrams taken from other processes around the larger company.

Then, I asked each of the six team members to sketch the process that they controlled together in shifts. Instead of receiving the anticipated six different flow diagrams, I received seven. One young operator was not certain, so she drew two!

We had an opportunity on our hands. We invited the head of engineering to visit the team and walk its members through the process to create a common understanding. It took a while, but that exercise led to a more uniform practice of process control. Essentially, it minimized the operator-to-operator variability. That, in turn, channeled more uniform product on to the subsequent unit operation, and so on through the entire process.

Similar sessions were carried out with each of the teams, and statistical tools appropriate to their segment of the process were introduced. Follow-up training was carried out by internal quality professionals with the motivation and support provided by George and the plant management.

Within 6 months, the subsidiary showed dramatic improvements in product quality and consumer satisfaction through increased process understanding and control. They retained their business with the company represented by my friend at the short course.

Eventually, because of their increased process knowledge, they grew in agility to the extent that they were able to produce specialty products, tailored for unique applications such as specialized pharmaceutical capsules and gelatin intended to support nail health. This, in turn, increased demand for their products, leading to increased profitability.

Discussion and key learnings

There are a number of lessons from this story. The first is that food products are not always used for food purposes - and gelatin is a prime example. Secondly, customers from outside the food industry may have different and much stricter requirements than food producers may be used to. Thirdly, this episode represents a safety crisis used for medical purposes, the presence of metal filings (already a food safety problem in its own right) became an acute threat to the X-ray procedures, with possibly very negative consequences for patients. Lastly, the safety crisis was a business crisis at the same time, with this gelatin representing a third of the company's business.

Fortunately, there are techniques and statistical tools that can be used in such situations and everywhere where companies seek to make their products more consistent, meet relevant specifications and improve overall quality.

Further reading

- Hoerl, R.W., Snee, R.D., 2020. Statistical Thinking: Improving Business Performance, third ed. John Wiley & Sons, Hoboken, NJ.
- Montgomery, D.C., 2013. Introduction to Statistical Quality Control, seventh ed. John Wiley and Sons, Hoboken, NJ.

Chapter Five

Hygienic design and cleaning

5.1 Managing Listeria: don't forget the human touch!

A cooked, sliced meats manufacturer in the UK in the early 1990s had a problem with Listeria monocytogenes (Lm). The counts in the finished product were always <100 cfu/g, but the incidence in product samples was high, approximately 5%. Typically, >300 finished product and >300 environmental samples were analyzed per month for Lm. Initial deep cleaning of the process lines and the high hygiene processing environment, together with more extensive dismantling of the slicers, to which the source of the Lm was traced (present on the slicer bed and gripper box), reduced the incidence of Lm in final product to approximately 1% but did not eliminate it. More investigations were needed to try and find any additional Lm sources.

Logs of meat, approximately 1m long and square shaped in profile, were sent to the slicing machine (Fig. 5.1.1) from the chilled store on a purpose-built trolley. The slicer operative picked up a log from the trolley, placed it on the bed of the slicer and then pressed the switch on the control panel to start slicing. After the log had been sliced, the log end was removed from the gripper box, discarded, another log was placed on the slicer bed and the cycle repeated itself. At the end of production, the control panel was quickly wiped over and covered in a plastic bag to protect it from the detergent foaming, rinsing and disinfectant application to the slicer. The slicer itself was appropriately dismantled and thoroughly cleaned and disinfected. Plastic protective covers were then removed from water sensitive parts of the machine, and it was prepped for production.

Further microbiological investigations were undertaken by increasing finished product samples and swabbing the slicing machines. Finished product sampling consisted of opening the finished product pack and cutting off (with scissors) two of the square shaped sliced meat corners, which were then placed in sampling fluid, and homogenised by stomaching to produce a sample for testing. Investigations found that Lm was not detected from finished product until those produced at about 16.00 h. Production ran from 06.00 to 22.00. Swab sampling of the slicer found no other Lm sources, but Lm was detected in the "slicer on" switch on the control panel. A drawing of the switch is shown in Fig. 5.1.2 (original switch) and Lm was found between the switch and the switch body-fluids leaked out from the switch body as the switch cylinder was pressed into it.

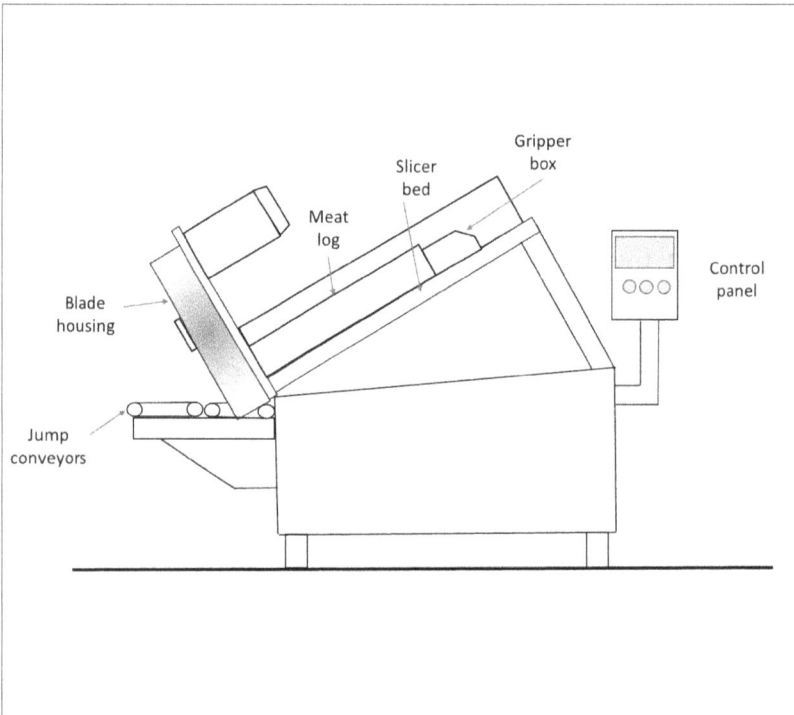

Fig 5.1.1: Schematic of the slicing machine and control panel.

The conclusion of the extended investigation proposed that Lm was present in the "on switch" on the control panel. The Lm was then transferred to the slicer operative's finger, then onto the log of meat (or gripper box) and then on to the bed of the slicer. There were probably only a few microorganisms transferred onto the operative's finger (the switch was not seen as a major, limitless source of Lm) and it was surmised that only by about 16.00 in the production day were there significant numbers of Lm on the slicer bed to be detected in finished product samples.

Following initial amendments to the cleaning and disinfection of the slicers in which further dismantling was undertaken prior to cleaning, the cleaning and disinfection program was further amended to include thorough cleaning and disinfection of the control panel with wipes before it was covered to allow the slicer to be cleaned. It was then wiped over again after the cover was removed.

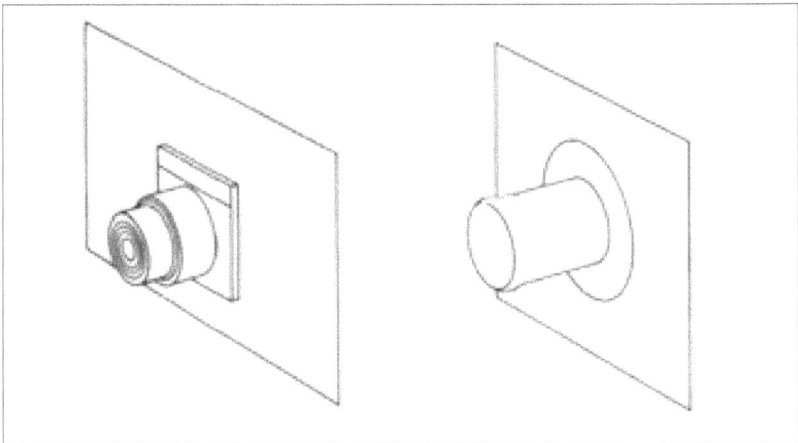

Fig 5.1.2: Schematic of the original switch in which Lm was found and a protective cover which could be purchased to help prevent fluid and particulate entry into the switch.

Schematic of the original switch in which Lm was found and a protective cover which could be purchased to help prevent fluid and particulate entry into the switch.

The design of the original switch was effectively uncleanable, but plastic protective covers were purchased to help make the switch design more hygienic.

Discussion and key learnings

The original reduction in prevalence of Lm in the finished product was the result of additional dismantling of the slicing machine until all surfaces where product could have contaminated were accessible for cleaning.

Manual interface points such as switches are equally as important as food contact surfaces and should be managed as such. They require a high degree of hygienic design and cleaning and disinfection. Ideally, they should be designed to not have crevices and dead spaces and more hygienic designs to aid cleanability are available, e.g., Fig. 5.1.3. The incident highlighted the inherent poor cleanability of some items of equipment with the only effective solution being redesign or replacement.

When microbiologically testing food products, always note the time of production. Detecting pathogens late in the production day may be indicative of a small pathogen source that needs time for growth and spread before cross-contamination can be detected. Alternatively, there may have been something happening in the plant at the initial time of Lm detection in product, e.g., a shift change, which could be a vector of cross-contamination.

As only two of the four corners of the finished product square slices were removed for microbiological testing, it was a lottery as to whether the corners of the log that actually sat on the bed of the slicer were chosen for analysis. In effect, there was a 50:50 chance that an Lm contaminated pack would be successfully identified, simply due to the way the sample was prepared for testing. Consideration should thus be given to the geometric relationship between the orientation of the product and product contact surfaces during production when deciding how to take product samples for testing. The sampling plan was subsequently changed so that whole meat slices were taken, homogenised and analyzed.

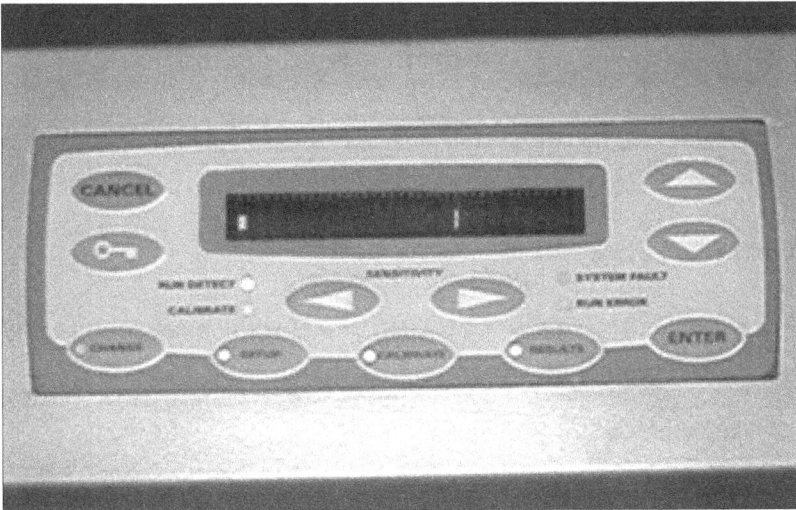

Fig 5.1.3: Hygienically designed control panel which can be easily cleaned.

Finally, lessons from hygienic design failures take a long time to be learnt and must be continually trained out to the food industry. Fig. 5.1.4 shows an image of a similar switch in 2015, 20 years after the first event, indicating the perfect conditions for Lm to be harbored, grow and be transferred to the operative's finger!

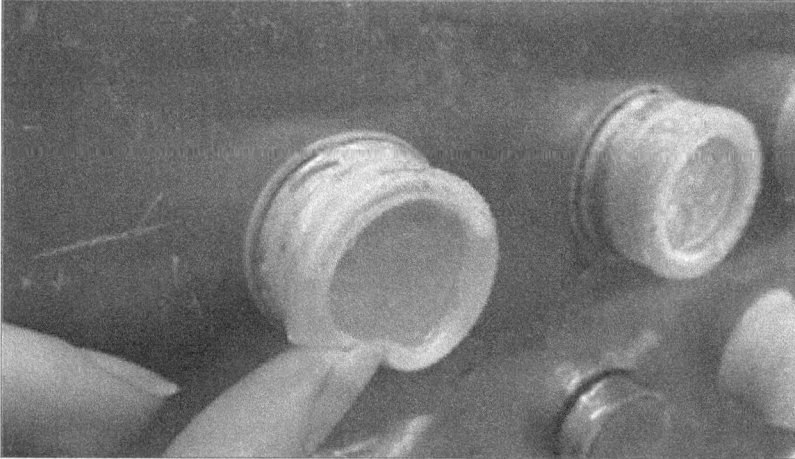

Fig 5.1.4: Fluid in switch provides an excellent potential Lm growth niche and transfer vector via operative's fingers.

Further reading

- AMI Sanitary Design Checklist. https://www.meatinstitute.org/index.php?ht¼a/GetDocument Action/i/7281.
- European Hygienic Engineering Design Group (EHEDG), 2018. Hygienic Design Principles.
- Guideline Document No. 8. John.Holah. /Downloads/. DOC_08_E_2018.pdf.
- EHEDG, 2004. Hygienic Design of Open Equipment for Processing of Food. Guideline Document No. 13. https://www.ehedg.org/guidelines/.

5.2 Plate heat exchanger as thermal insulator

An ice cream factory had to shut down because of persistent high microbial counts in the final product, despite the pasteurization of the ice cream mix.

The design of the process line looked correct and the line had been running for a long time without microbiological problems. It was built from hygienic components, but the microbial counts of the pasteurized product started increasing and reached an unacceptable level. The cause was a mystery. Inspection of the process line down from the plate heat exchanger (PHE) did not show anything wrong and the microbial counts of the ingoing unpasteurized product were not higher than usual. It was concluded that the PHE itself must be the cause of the problem. It was decided to clean the PHE two times before production and also to "pre-pasteurize" the line twice before resuming production. Amazingly, this did not improve the microbial results and after a week of trying, production of ice cream was halted. That was the state of affairs when I was invited.

Having seen the microbial counts and the inspection reports of the process line, I asked why they had not opened the PHE for inspection. The indignant response was that a PHE should never be taken apart. It was explained to me that during the process of disassembling the PHE, there would be a risk of damaging the rubber seals between the plates, which then would cause severe problems and the factory would have to bring in the manufacturer of the PHE to reassemble it. The staff felt certain that the PHE was clean after two times cleaning-in-place (CIP) before every production. As they unsuccessfully tried every possible troubleshooting option, I suggested that perhaps the denatured protein had formed a layer of deposit on the plates of the PHE. That deposit would then act as a thermal insulation and the heating control system would automatically increase the temperature of the heating medium to ensure that the temperature set for the pasteurization would be reached. As a result, more protein would build up and the problem would get worse. Eventually, but reluctantly, they disassembled the PHE.

To their unpleasant surprise, the product side of the PHE was not clean at all. The plates were covered by a layer of a quite solid dark brown substance. The layer of brownish substance did not only act as a thermal insulator, it was actually so thick that the gap between the plates was significantly reduced. As a result, the volume between the plates was reduced, the velocity of the product between the plates became higher, and the effective pasteurization time became shorter. In other words, the PHE did not pasteurize correctly. Although the records showed that the correct temperature was reached, the residence time needed for pasteurization was insufficient.

After looking at the design of the PHE, it could be concluded that the cross section of the space between the plates was about four times larger than the cross section of the adjacent pipelines. Because the flow rate for CIP of the line was based on the cross section of the pipeline, the velocity of the cleaning liquid in the PHE was far too low to provide a necessary turbulent flow to adequately clean.

The problem was solved by using a separate circuit for CIP of the PHE, increasing the flow rate to reach the 1.5 m/s velocity needed for effective cleaning. I have seen similar problems in various dairy plants and every time increasing the flow rate solved the problem.

Discussion and key learnings

- Never assume that equipment is clean if that cannot be directly observed. A mechanical difficulty is not a reason for not inspecting the product side of the equipment, in particular, if there is an unexplained problem.
- Base the flow rate for CIP not only on the cross section of the piping used but also on the cross section of other components of the process line, be it a PHE, valves, or anything else.
- Using a PHE, monitoring the temperature of the product is not sufficient. Monitoring the temperature of the heating medium is equally important. If the temperature of the heating medium goes up, something must be wrong with the heat transfer.

Further reading

Goode, K.R., Christian, G.K., Fryer, P.J., 2016. Improving the cleaning of heat exchangers. In: Lelieveld, H., Holah, J., Gabrić, D. (Eds.), Handbook of Hygiene Control in the Food Industry, second ed., pp. 465-489.

5.3 Aseptic flow meter in a dairy cream line

A new process line for sterilizing dairy cream, to be followed by aseptic packaging, had been operating for less than a week when the aseptically packed products appeared not to be sterile. All packs that were produced about an hour after the start of the production were contaminated.

Even if the sterilization of the packs before filling would not always be 100%, it was felt that the aseptic-packing machine could not be responsible for the massive contamination. Firstly, the packaging line was built from high-quality hygienic and bacteria-tight components. Secondly, every time the production stopped, the line was cleaned and sterilized again. Third, after the cleaning-in-place (CIP) process, the line was thoroughly inspected. Each time, the inspection showed that all components were perfectly clean and should not affect the pre-sterilization. Still, the product got contaminated.

Because of the rejection of tons of cream every day, the problem became extremely and unsustainably expensive. What was expected to be a profit-making new product had turned into a nightmare.

When I arrived to assist finding the cause of the problem, initially I could not find anything wrong with the process line. All components looked fine and clean after CIP and none of the components showed any obvious leak.

Nevertheless, the microorganisms in the product must have come from somewhere. Hence, the logical next step was to look for less obvious sources of leaks. Near the end of the pipeline to the packaging machine, there was an electromagnetic flow meter. In principle, this should have been an ideal design for aseptic process lines, because basically it was just a pipe section with some electronics around it. To be able to measure the flow rate, however, two electrodes had to be in contact with the product that was flowing through the device. The electrodes had to be electrically insulated from the steel pipe section.

Upon inspection, it was found that the two tiny (about 4 mm ⌀) electrodes were mounted almost completely flat within the inside of the pipe and were insulated with tiny rings made from easily cleanable polytetrafluoroethylene (PTFE) that at the same time served as the barrier seal between the inside and the outside of the pipe. Although a leak could not be observed, it was decided to open the tight housing of the device that protected the electronics against moisture. There appeared to be several millilitres of cream inside the housing, which could only have come through the electrode seal construction. The leak, however, was so small that it had taken quite some time for the cream to penetrate from the pipe into the housing. Once there, the bacteria could multiply in the cream. The leak was big enough to let the bacteria pass back in the other direction, from the housing to the product side. When the inside of the product pipe was thoroughly cleaned, it took the bacteria inside the housing of the electronics apparently just about an hour to get back into the product stream and contaminate it.

During sterilization of the line before the start of the production, the thermal expansion of the PTFE seal rings, clamped between metal parts (the steel pipe and the platinum electrodes), caused the shape of the PTFE rings to change. It could be calculated that this was enough to create a gap of about 10-20 µm between the metal and the PTFE rings. This was more than enough for the passage of microorganisms that are less than 1 µm in size. Such a small gap is virtually impossible to observe during inspection because the amount of liquid passing the gap may be just microliters per hour. After cleaning the housing and replacing the PTFE rings by resilient synthetic rubber rings, the microbiological problem was solved and production could be resumed, now successfully.

Discussion and key learnings

- Never give up if nothing can be seen, because the eye cannot see everything. Persist until the cause of the problem is found. There always is a cause.
- Never use PTFE in food processing lines, it does not provide a reliable seal. In whatever way mounted in an equipment, it will create crevices that will harbor microorganisms that are protected against cleaning and disinfection.
- Select food processing equipment, including measuring devices, that have no PTFE components.
- This case shows limits of the efficacy of visual inspections or audits.

Further reading

Lelieveld, H.L.M., Holah, J., 2016. Specific requirements for equipment for aseptic processing. In: Lelieveld, H., Holah, J., Gabric, D. (Eds.), Handbook of Hygiene Control in the Food Industry, pp. 389-394.

5.4 Lessons learned from a contamination investigation

I worked as a plant hygienist at a nutritional products manufacturer where comprehensive cleaning and sanitation procedures and environmental monitoring programs were in place.

Once, the microbiology lab reported the growth of mold in the test samples. A considerable quantity of product was rejected. The cross-department investigation team worked hard to find the source of mold and the root cause(s). The dried powder product was stored in silos, transported along the powder transfer lines, and packed in the respective fillers. The team studied the sequence of production, the configuration of silos, and transfer lines. All suspected areas were opened and cleaned up. The mold growth seemed to disappear. After a few weeks, the mold appeared again. Many tons of products were rejected.

After several rounds of brainstorming and thorough inspection of the area, further investigation narrowed down the source to mainly two silos. But the trouble was finding where precisely the mold was growing. The investigation team felt that all places that could support mold growth had already been investigated, cleaned up, and verified. There was only one area left unopened, and that was the belt that was wrapped around the place where the cylindrical body and the conical discharge of the silo were joined. The belt was there to absorb the vibration while filling or emptying the silo. Finally, the team decided to detach the belt from the silo surface. Removing the belt was tough at first because we did not have the right tools. Once removed, it was confirmed that the mold growth was happening in between the stainless-steel surface and the rubber belt. Later, proper tools were fabricated and silo cleaning, sanitation, and verification procedures were revised. Once the cause was eliminated, the contamination stopped.

We found that released products had not been compromised, but there had been huge quantities rejected and very significant costs involved for cleaning, sanitation, and verification in this episode.

Discussion and key learnings

1. Involve all related departments in investigating the source of the problem production, engineering, and QA/QC are vital departments in the investigation.
2. Open communication and respecting everyone's opinion is critical in narrowing down to the causes of the problem. While the quality personnel have expertise in identifying the microorganisms and how they grow, operators and maintenance technicians know the equipment inside out. Combining expertise from all departments was the key to a successful investigation.
3. Pay full attention to the hygienic design of the equipment. Do not assume all possible areas are investigated when the results show that contamination still continues.
4. Focus on the investigation - the costs of dismantling, cleaning, verification, and reassembling were high. Still, if you try to save in the investigative phase, you may incur higher costs of rejects later, or the problem may even lead to recall if minute mold colonies get into the product.
5. Do not get complacent on the existing cleaning, sanitation, and verification programs. Conduct regular reviews of effectiveness.
6. In addition to the measures above, after an incident, investigate the consequences for the food safety system

that might (should) have prevented this from happening in the first place. Was hygienic design a part of the overall risk assessment of the plant? Is there a comprehensive cleaning/sanitation plan?

Are plant employees sufficiently trained? Are responsibilities clearly defined? Are instructions clear? Is there enough time scheduled for maintenance and cleaning? All these questions (and the above list is probably not exhaustive) involve management responsibility for developing, implementing, and maintaining the overall food safety system.

Further reading

Motarjemi, Y., Wallace, C.A., 2014. Incident management and root cause analysis. In: Motarjemi, Y., Lelieved, H. (Eds.), Food Safety Management: A Practical Guide for the Food Industry. Academic Press. Waltham MA, pp 1017-1036

5.5 "Superhygienic", very expensive membrane valve

A processing line for sterile milk appeared to be impossible to sterilize even if the temperature was increased to ever higher levels and with absurdly long sterilization times. After a short time of operation, the milk always appeared to be contaminated.

It was a new line with the best available components, all of aseptic design, including a magnetically driven and bacteria-tight centrifugal pump, approved aseptic couplings and aseptic diaphragm valves recently designed, and the pride of the valve manufacturer. The cleaning-in-place process was well designed. No residual dirt could be detected anywhere. After the sterilization process, the line should have been sterile and could not be the cause of the problem.

Asked to assist in solving the problem, I demanded to literally take every component apart. That meant the pump, the couplings, and the valves. The static seal of the pump housing, the seals of all the hygienic couplings, all were in perfect condition. The only potential culprit left was the valves. However, after opening, the first valve looked perfectly clean and it had indeed a beautifully white smooth polytetrafluoroethylene (PTFE) diaphragm. Hence, there was no need for a lip seal as used in valves in process lines before the sterilization step. Then, tools were brought in to remove all parts of the first valve. When the diaphragm came loose, suddenly there was such a disgusting smell that everybody watching jumped away.

Clearly, the diaphragm that was intended to prevent any connection from the inside of the valve with the outside had failed. Upon close inspection, it appeared that a tiny amount of rotten milk was present on the circumference of the connection between the metal housing and the diaphragm. No microbiological analysis was needed to prove the spoilage of the tiny amount of milk trapped between the diaphragm rim and the steel. Then, the second valve, same type, was taken apart, and everybody was careful not to be too close with their nose to the valve. We found the same there. The valves did not conform with their hygienic design.

PTFE looks nice and hygienic and it has splendid properties. If the manufacturing process is right, it can be easy to clean and to inspect for cleanliness. However, a disadvantage that the valve designer had overlooked was that PTFE has very little resilience. If clamped between steel surfaces, there will be a tight seal. During sterilization of the line, the PTFE is heated (in the tests even to >135◦C) and expands. After cooling, it shrinks. Then, the seal no longer lives up to its name. The milk that had entered into the capillary space during earlier use of the line allowed the multiplication of bacteria in that space. Only one bacterium is needed to completely contaminate the tiny amount of milk after less than a day. The PTFE protected the anaerobic spoilage bacteria, well known for their appalling smell, against the sterilization temperature. Again, one of those bacteria is enough to recontaminate the process line after sterilization.

In discussion with the manufacturer, the design was changed by adding a synthetic rubber ring between the diaphragm and the steel housing. The resilient rubber compensated the lack of resilience of the PTFE. Indeed, after this modification the problem did not reoccur. The manufacturer then permanently changed the design.

Discussion and key learnings

- PTFE looks nice but cannot be used as a sealing material. After heating, its dimensions change enough to create invisible but real passages for the <1 μm size bacteria.
- Manufacturers offering components for aseptic process lines should have their designs tested for sterilizability and bacteria tightness prior to selling them.

5.6 Feeling the heat with Escherichia coli (periodically)

Sandwiches produced with ingredient fillings made on a large industrial mixer were contaminated with Escherichia coli. Only sandwiches containing ingredients prepared on the mixer were contaminated suggesting there was a source of E. coli within the machine. Batches made immediately after cleaning the mixer were more likely to be contaminated and the mixer was a heavily used machine.

Operatives were noted to be overfilling the machine with ingredients for mixing.

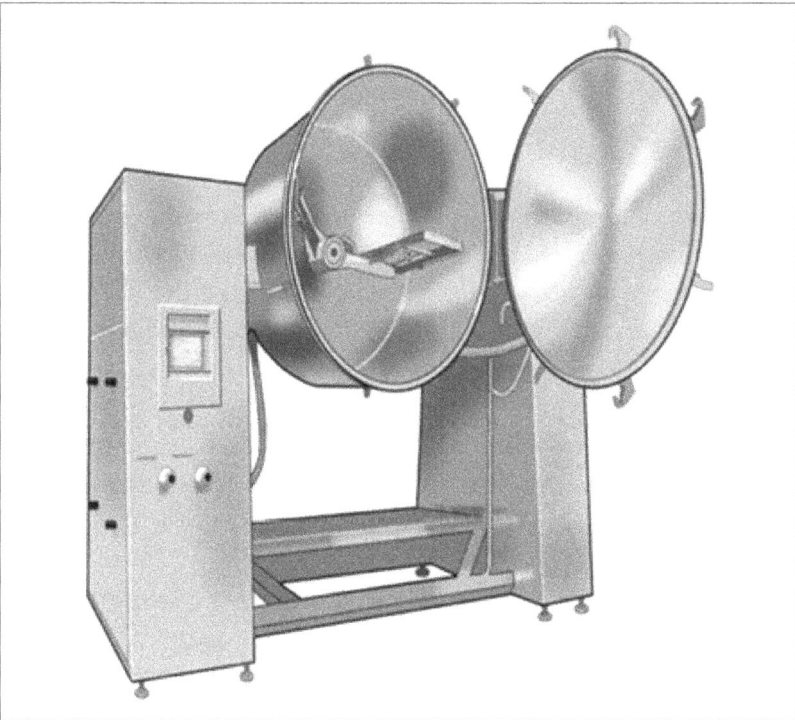

Schematic industrial mixer showing mixing paddle on drive shaft.

However, the actual cleaning and disinfection of the mixer was very good with no indications of hygiene indicator failings using adenosine triphosphate and total viable count microbial sampling.

E. coli was not expected to be a problem in this area of the factory as the room temperature and ingredients were chilled and the minimum growth temperature for E. coli is approximately 7 to 8°C, considerably higher than, e.g., Listeria (approximately 1°C) usually associated with chilled, ready-to-eat products.

The food manufacturer experimented with a number of different detergents, disinfectants, and cleaning frequencies for both interim and end-of-production cleaning, but little success was achieved in reducing the E. coli incidence in product.

Further investigations found that the source of the E. coli was in the recess around the shaft seal and behind this into the bearing/drive motor area. The overloading of the mixer with product leading to excess weight in the vessel added stress to the drive shaft and mixing paddles making it move excessively in the recess. This allowed food products to collect in this area. Over time, the movement caused the seal to be damaged and therefore allowed product to seep into the recess and into the bearing/drive motor behind the shaft and seal.

When the mixer was cleaned and disinfected, the surfaces of the mixer were visually clean. However, when the machine restarted, all the debris that had seeped into the rear of the machine seeped back through into the main vessel and mixed with (primarily) the first product batch leading to contaminated product.

The use of a thermal imaging camera showed that the surface temperature of the mixer around the shaft area was higher than the rest of the equipment.

The conclusion of the extended investigation proposed that food soils were able to push into the shaft seal area and beyond the seal into the bearing/drive motor area.

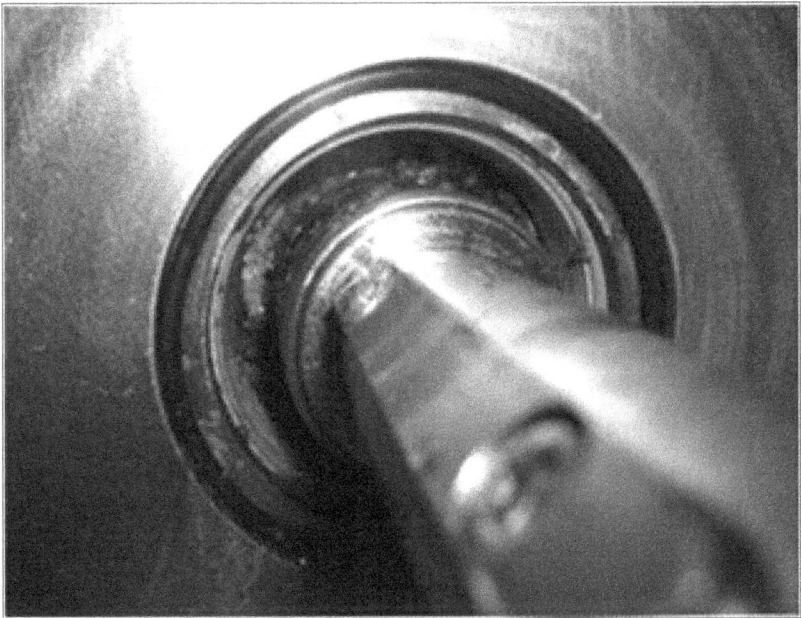

Build-up of contamination in the mixer shaft seal area.

The soil provided a growth medium for the E. coli, which was able to grow in the chilled conditions because friction from the drive shaft locally increased temperatures in this area of the equipment, sufficient for E. coli to grow.

Control was reinstated by introducing routine full strip downs of the machine with deep cleaning and regular seal checks and replacement. These cleaning procedures were in addition to the normal within-production (interim) and end-of-production cleans and were known as periodic cleans. Cleaning instruction cards (CICs), also known as sanitary standard operation procedures (SSOPs), were then revised to incorporate the three cleans prescribed for the equipment: interim, end-of-production, and periodic.

The mixer was also no longer overloaded, also effectively extending the life of the shaft seals.

Discussion and key learnings

Changes in cleaning chemicals and disinfectants, which will have been initially chosen for their performance in controlling the specific soiling conditions associated with the equipment and its products and appear to be still working as intended, will generally have little effect on microbiological incidents. Cleaning chemical changes per se is not the answer: a source and/or vector of the microbial contamination has to be found. The local generation of heat in items of equipment may allow the proliferation of microbial flora not associated with growth in ostensibly chilled conditions more suited to psychrotrophs. Higher local temperatures may also lead to more rapid growth of the psychrotrophs (such as Listeria) more likely to be found in these environments. Some indication of "hot spots" in equipment can be found by looking at equipment surface temperatures with infrared cameras.

Poor practices associated with the use of machines (in this case excessive product loading) may have impacts on the fabric of the machine leading to enhanced microbial harbourage.

If the first product batch manufactured after cleaning is primarily contaminated, this often suggests failures in the cleaning and disinfection program. Using this concept, the testing of the first product from a cleaned machine, when microorganisms may be exposed by the movements of the machine when it is switched on, is a useful microbial investigation tool.

Food production machinery, particularly those used for the manufacture of ready-to-eat (RTE) food products, should be assessed for any issues related to hygienic design such as rotating shafts and seals, dead areas where product soils could accumulate beyond the reach of cleaning fluids, and metal-to-metal joints which could harbor microorganisms. On the basis of this risk assessment, a frequency of periodic cleans should be established where, over and above end-of-production cleaning, the machine can be dismantled to a degree where all areas in which soils and microorganisms could penetrate to are exposed for cleaning and disinfection.

Finally, templates for CICs or SSOPs should be divided into sections for interim, end-of-production, and periodic cleaning to focus attention to the hygiene manager to assess the need for periodic practices. In the experience of the author, the lack of periodic cleaning practices in the RTE food sector has been responsible for many food pathogen contamination issues and any education and training in this area can only be beneficial.

Further reading

- AMI Sanitary design checklist. https://www.meatinstitute.org/index.php?ht=a/GetDocumentAction/i/7281
- Holah, J.T., 2014. Cleaning and disinfection practices in food processing. In: Lelieveld, H.L.M., Holah, J., Napper, D. (Eds.), Hygiene in Food Processing: Principles and Practice, second ed. Woodhead Publishing Limited. ISBN 978-0-85709-429-2.

5.7 Listeria in grated cheese

At lunch with a friend, we came to talk about events and problems at our workplaces. He was the production manager of a cheese production company at the time and told me that for a few weeks he had been having problems with Listeria monocytogenes, which was now being detected more and more frequently in the grated cheese they produced.

He explained to me that the cheese the company produced was made partly from their own production and partly bought from other suppliers. As the company had a monitoring program for Listeria for their own production, he assumed that the contamination was coming from the supplied cheeses. However, he had never detected Listeria in the cheeses supplied to him. I asked him about his cleaning plan and whether the cleaning was validated. At the word validation, he just looked at me in amazement indicating that he did not know what validation was. We agreed that I would take a closer look with my team.

At the agreed time, we met in the production plant at the end of the working day. After the end of production, all machines were carefully cleaned, disassembled where necessary, and disinfected. When this was finished, the last step was to clean the floor with a high-pressure cleaner. This involved spraying a lot of water back onto the clean equipment. Analytically, we could confirm that the cheese used, the cleaned equipment, and tools were free of Listeria, but the high-pressure cleaning of the floor recontaminated the production equipment with this pathogen and we found it in the drainage of the floor.

Discussion and key learnings

Insufficient knowledge about the ecology and characteristics of L. monocytogenes led to a failure of this company to recognize that their cleaning plan was wrongly designed. Listeria is an environmental bacterium that can be very easily introduced into a food production facility, where it can survive and multiply. Residual water and drains are known reservoirs for the pathogen. Therefore, using a high-pressure cleaner for the floor at the end of a cleaning program is absolutely prohibited, because it will spray a lot of dirt and droplets, which then settle on all surfaces that are not protected.

In case of heavy soiling, these surfaces must be cleaned first, and this includes the floor. Then the production equipment can be cleaned. Finally, the floor is gently cleaned. In addition, the effectiveness of the cleaning must be validated on a regular predefined basis and be supported by ongoing Listeria monitoring to demonstrate that the cleaning plan and all cleaning methods lead to the specified results.

Further reading

- Handbook of Hygiene Control in the Food Industry. Chapter 6: Aerosols as a Contamination Risk, 2016. Elsevier.
- Ryther, R., 2014. Development of a comprehensive cleaning and sanitizing program for food production facilities (Chapter 27). In: Motarjemi, Y., Lelieveld, H. (Eds.), Food Safety Management, a Practical Guide for Food Industry. Elsevier.

5.8 Microbiological problems with a meat processing line

A meat factory in North America, belonging to a multinational company, had a persistent microbiological problem and had to reject many of the sausages produced for several weeks in a row. They had manually cleaned the pumps and valves and "sterilized" the entire process line several times before starting production, but nothing seemed to work. They had checked the process conditions and found them to be correct, every time. They were desperate. The local official food safety inspector agreed that they had done all they could, but nevertheless many batches had to be rejected. That was the moment that management felt they had to inform the parent company, and I was asked to go and find out what the problem was.

Seeing nothing wrong with the records, I went to inspect the offending process line after cleaning and asked for various components, such as the valves and pumps now cleaned manually, to be dismantled. Indeed, they looked clean and moreover they were of correct design, with no crevices and dead areas. Following the process line, in a long section of a straight pipe, I discovered a socket for a remote temperature sensor. It happened to be on a short "T". I asked to take it apart, but the employees seemed reluctant. It was essential for the compulsory temperature recording and was of hygienic design, but it had been difficult to get it to work. They much preferred to leave it as it is. The head of the department, the engineering department, and also the inspector all agreed that taking it apart would cause more problems, not less. Things were escalated to the local director, who finally agreed to my request, as he didn't want to go against advice from the parent company.

The small "hygienic temperature sensor" was disconnected and we found it full of semisolid product debris. And so, the problem was identified and from then onwards the socket was dismantled and manually cleaned before sanitation. The problem was solved.

Discussion and key learnings

- Do not assume that a hygienically designed process line is always cleanable in place.
- If inspecting a process line, don't make assumptions. That is never assume that some components may be left out of the inspection scheme because they "cannot be the cause of a problem."
- Make sure you really understand the problem yourself, before supporting other people's opinions.

Further reading

Lelieveld, H.L.M., 1976. Influence of stagnant areas in process equipment on the increase of microorganism concentrations in the product: a tentative mathematical approach. Biotechnol. Bioeng. 18, 1807-1810.

5.9 Spoilage of UHT-milk

One morning in the late 1990s, I was called by the production manager of the largest dairy plant in the region and asked to attend a meeting as soon as possible. Also present were a representative of the manufacturer of the aseptic filling line and one of the largest retailers in the country. They reported to me that during the monitoring of a UHT-milk, they found a heavy contamination with coliforms from time to time. Upon further investigation, they identified the bacteria to be Enterobacter sakazakii.

The contamination was very irregular and affected about 5 packs out of 10,000 and the retailer threatened to take the dairy off their list if the contamination level could not be reduced to 1 in 10,000. This was the triggering point for the dairy to take action, although, as I later learned, it had already had complaints from consumers for some time that the UHT-milk was spoiling before the expiry date. As they did not find the reason for the defect in their own finished product analyses, no action was taken.

Our investigations in cooperation with technicians from the aseptic filling company revealed that the weld seam was not perfectly parallel when the container was formed and therefore leaks occurred in a few packs, although no milk was visibly leaking out. In addition, the conveyor belt between the filling station and the final packaging in four packs was not clean. Between the links of the metal conveyor belt, there was a significant biofilm, containing high levels of E. sakazakii.

Packs would remain on this conveyor belt until they were sealed in foils, and while the conveyor belt continued to run, it spread the biofilm onto the underside of the milk packs. If a package had a defective weld, contamination could occur.

Discussion and key learnings

A combination of several faults led to this event. First of all, there was insufficient maintenance of the equipment, especially of the packaging equipment, to detect the bad weld seam of the package in time. This has to be done by ongoing careful inspection of packs on a random basis.

For a long period, the conveyor belt was insufficiently cleaned; therefore, a massive biofilm was formed. It is hence recommended that the cleaning program of equipment to be designed based on the evaluation of the risks of contamination. Consumer complaints are an important indicator in any food safety and quality management system. This was not treated seriously enough here. There was a misconception that any contamination could be found through end-product testing, which was completely wrong, because the contamination did not occur regularly and to such a small extent that it could not be detected through end-product analysis. The consumer complaints should have led to hygiene checks in the plant, and so the biofilm would have been found. In that case, the defective sealing of the milk packs would probably also have been found.

Side note: This story occurred in the late 1990s when E. sakazakii was not yet known as a serious pathogen. At that time, this bacterium belonged to the coliforms and was one of the indicator organisms. For us, it was ideal for revealing the contamination route. With today's knowledge, the action and reaction of those responsible for production must be completely different: stop production, investigate which lots are affected, possibly recall them, and investigate the cause of the contamination in more depth.

Further reading

- Götz, A., Wani, A.A., Langowski, H.-C., Wunderlich, J., 2014. Aseptic packaging. In: Motarjemi, Y., Moy, G., Todd, E. (Eds.), Encyclopaedia of Food Safety, vol. 3. Elsevier, pp. 124-134.
- Hygienic Design of Belt Conveyors for the Food Industry. EHEDG-Guideline 43, 2016. www. ehedg.org/guidelines/.

5.10 Mold problems

A low-fat spreads manufacturing site, part of a larger conglomerate, in an industrialized country in Asia had been struggling with mold problems for some time. Central company specialists - microbiologists, packaging technicians, sanitation, and hygienic design engineers - had been working with the site to eliminate all possible causes. They had worked with the supplier of the tubs and lids, for which they also introduced additional cleaning procedures at the site; they removed all supplier-related pallets and secondary (corrugated board) packaging material from the production hall, put all workers through stricter personal hygiene training, upgraded the workers' uniforms so they looked more like hazmat suits, carried out a deep cleaning of the line and surroundings, and installed plastic curtains around the line in order to assure a laminar flow of filtered air. Finally, they installed an airlock at the main entrance and closed off all other entrances. Before getting into the production area, people now needed to get into a lock and be "showered" with ultraclean air for a minute before being released to the other side. This applied to everybody - workers, maintenance technicians, contractors, management. Things got somewhat better, but the problem was not entirely solved.

Then an audit team visited the factory. Naturally, they had to see the production hall, so they put on the special "hazmat" suits and lined up before the airlock. The first auditor went through, waiting for his colleagues to be air-showered, and looked around. Around 5 m from the airlock, there appeared to be a door in the wall. He went to the door, turned the handle, and found himself back in the hallway where the rest of the audit team and representatives of plant management were waiting their turn to pass through the lock. The plant manager appeared utterly shocked and said he had never known this door existed and people could simply walk in and out, bypassing the time-consuming airlock procedure. Subsequent interviews revealed that workers and maintenance people felt that the airlock was too much of a hassle and doubted whether this was really necessary, so they unlocked this (previously closed off) bypass. This appeared to be silently condoned by the management.

Afterward, the door was permanently and irreversibly closed; this whole episode had personal consequences for the management and the site got their mold problems under control under new management.

Discussion and key learnings

It is the attitude of local management and the local culture it creates for employees, much more than the general level of industrialization in the country, which ultimately makes or breaks all food safety and quality systems (the best run manufacturing site this author has seen on his travels around the world was located in the middle of nowhere in a "developing" country in another part of the world). While the mold problem was a technical problem in itself, getting a grip on the problem required the awareness and commitment of local management. While that was lacking, all technical efforts ultimately fell short and it took a change of local leadership to bring the problems under control.

Chapter Six

Auditing

6.1 Audit tales

I used to be a food safety auditor for Global Food Safety Initiative (GFSI) standards, specifically BRC Food and FSSC 22,000. One of my typical audit activities was to assess control records from the preceding 2 or 3 months to identify trends and inconsistencies. Based on such experiences, I will share some revealing evidence of human creativity and the importance of process verification. These stories are all different, but they also have fundamental things in common, so there will be one paragraph with learnings and conclusions at the end.

Case 1: very steady temperature log

Assessing some manually written temperature logs, I realized that the figures were always the same for a cold room: 5.0; 5.0; 5.0∘C . for hours, days, weeks and months!

So, I decided to see the cold room and interview the operator personally. Mr. Pedro, who maintained and signed the records that I had seen, was working that shift.

The audit happened some years ago, and the thermometer was a traditional analogue instrument . and it showed 5.0∘C exactly!!! Even when the door opened during a loading operation, the thermometer reading did not fluctuate. Then I talked to the operator:

- Mr. Pedro, I know you have been working in this position for a long time, and I observed the temperature is very steady in this room. Could you please let me know how it is possible?
- Yes, lady. Some time ago, the company owner said if we do not pass the audit, all employees will lose their jobs. And

this room is a critical step of our process, so the records must always be at 5 degrees, and we shall put all efforts to keep this value. So, my colleagues and I decided to fix two pins to hold the pointer in the right position.

Case 2: chlorine and pH level

During one audit, a manual record of water quality, specifically chlorine intake and pH, showed a suspicious trend: narrow results variations. The most frequent result was 6.1 . 6.1 .. 6.1 .. sometimes 7.0 .. The chlorine levels appeared to be reasonable and showing more normal fluctuations.

I decided to see the pH meter and one "live" measurement. The laboratory technician rapidly brought me stripes. How was it possible to have a result like 6.1 using strips ranging from zero to 14, only whole numbers, no fractions?

- Could you please measure the water pH at this moment? I asked.
- Of course, the result is 6.0!
- Great, what you do in this case?
- -Well, the ideal pH is from 6.5 to 7.5. So as it is below the target, we must correct the value by adding an alkaline solution to the water reservoir.
- Tell me a little bit about it. Is there a working procedure for it?
- Yes, there is (opening a folder). See here: "in case the pH is below 7.0, add 1 liter of an alkaline solution to the tank. If you could please follow me? I will do this right now.

He did his job correctly at this point. But the question remained:

- Why can we see in the records values like 6.1 if you use a stripe.

- I can explain we got six from the stripe result. Now I add a comma after the number six to document I have added 1 litre of the solution in the tank.

I realized his boss, who was observing everything, blushed immediately.

Case 3: rinse water

I was at a fruit juice processor, more specifically, UHT packed products. It is part of the daily routine of this product category to check rinse water pH to confirm no residues remain after CIP cleaning.

During the traceability assessment, still in the site quality office, I realized that although this parameter was a labeled as a CCP, there was no history of deviation at all. I reviewed more than 4 months back, and the pH was always according to the specifications.

Of course, based on previous experiences, I decided to talk to the operators to understand the "magic" behind these "perfect" results.

The operator seemed to be very qualified and knowledgeable about his job and the control's importance. He was able to explain what to do in case of very low or very high pH value on rinse water: to repeat rinsing with pure water. So, I asked him directly:

- Do you work here in this position already for a long time? - Yes, more than 10 years.
- Is the pH always stable or do you experience variations?
- Well, the pH is relatively stable, but more or less one or two times a week, we have deviations.

- Thanks for the information. I have not seen any data in the logs showing the deviations or any information in the corrective action field. How are they recorded?
- Lady, you will never see deviations on my records. When I get a bad result, I only repeat the rinsing and measure the pH again and again until to get the RIGHT result.

And he said again: You will never see a deviation documented on my records, only the right result.

Case 4: manual food labeling

This case is not related to audit logs, but is very current topic, especially with new GFSI requirements on un-announced audits.

In the beginning of my career, my first customers were great malls, and I was contracted to inspect food court restaurants. My presence was not exactly welcome, but the business owners had to accept our "visit" by order of the mall administrator.

One day, I had to carry out an un-announced audit to prevent a cover-up of the "crime scene" in anticipation of my visit.

As a background: in these restaurants, small batches are usually prepared in advance, in individual portions, packed into plastic bags. Furthermore, according to our regulation, all portioned food shall be labeled (even manually) with expiration date and traceability data.

I found all bags with no identification in the refrigerator. And I asked: Hello guys. Tell me, why are these food bags not labeled?

I did not know you would come today, lady!

Case 5: the Lenin medal

During an audit in an Eastern European country, where my company had just acquired a manufacturing site after the iron curtain had come down, I checked temperature controls and found a very simple household thermometer, hanging from the ceiling by a piece of rope, in the middle of what was supposed to be a temperature-controlled warehouse. For answers to the question whether this thermometer was calibrated and what the records showed, I was referred to a lady who was in charge of all records. The walls of her office were packed with binders, with records going back ages. My little thermometer, however, was nowhere to be found in the records. When asked about this omission, she said that simple thermometers hanging by a piece of rope didn't qualify. In order to be part of the official record, it had to be a "serious instrument". My objection that it was not so much what the instrument looked like, but whether it played an important role in the temperature chain of the product, was dismissed. She had some 30 years in this position, and I would have to agree that she knew the plant and the systems better than I did. When I mentioned that this would be a non-conformity, she responded that she had received the Lenin medal for QA and the discussion ended there. At a follow-up visit, the hanging thermometer had been replaced by a "serious instrument" and temperatures were being properly recorded.

Discussion and key learnings

This is all about people, how they interpret what is expected of them, how they try to do a good job and take pride in that, and how they deal with things that don't make sense to them. The stories show that just telling people what to do and what the expected results are is not enough and may sometimes be counterproductive. They need to understand not only the "what" but also the "why".

- Always explain the reason behind an instruction and do not threaten people into taking desperate measures. It is a fundamental element of food safety culture.
- Never let the operators associate poor results on logs with poor performance on their jobs.
- Spend some time with your team in the laboratory to understand how they should interpret results, not only how do they perform the tests.
- Explain that food safety requirements should be met at all times, not just a preparation for an audit.
- Take the time and invest in education in order to properly integrate a new acquisition, which may have operated a very different food safety culture for a long time.

6.2 Wing nuts and a blow torch

I was working as a field inspector for the Department of Agriculture, visiting a dairy company. On this one assignment, I was to inspect a midsize cheese factory for its cheese manufacturing and whey processing operations. The plant had not been inspected previously and my task was to assess the condition, sanitation, and cleaning of equipment.

As I was investigating the operations, I heard a loud clanging sound coming from the front area of the cheese vats. Investigating the noise, I found the plant manager hammering on the wing nuts securing the face plate of a small positive displacement pump. This was used to move the whey from the cheese vats for future processing.

I advised the plant manager that his efforts were no longer necessary. I would record the pump as unsatisfactory as the interior of the installation could not be inspected. I also advised that he should continue the operation but replace the pump and open it in the maintenance shop.

He replied, "No, you asked to see it and I'll make sure you do." It was his decision, so I continued my inspection elsewhere. Eventually the clanging stopped so I returned to the area. At this point the plant manager was using an acetylene torch to cut the bolts from the face plate. A heavy swing of the hammer sent the faceplate skittering across the floor. A thick green slime started to drip from the rear seal area behind the pump lobes.

The plant manager, a quick thinker, said, "Well, it didn't come apart that hard yesterday!"

Discussion and key learnings

The plant manager's statement was obviously true. The pump had not been disassembled the day before or for many days before. Too often plant personnel take the concept of clean-in-place (CIP) to mean they don't have to do daily inspections of cleaning, gaskets, and seals. Secondly, the positive displacement pump was not designed for CIP cleaning even though it was situated in a CIP pipeline circuit and, therefore, needed special attention.

The fact that this pump, that was not properly maintained and severely soiled, was contaminating all the whey that passed through it made this situation especially critical.

6.3 Poisonous patisserie (or why management attitude determines safe food)

I was auditing a bakery supplier with a colleague. The company also produced patisserie containing fresh cream. The premises were not well organized, and the flow was not logical. Procedures to prevent cross-contamination did not exist and cream was not whipped in a chilled environment. As we examined the cream processing, we noticed that the use by date (it was pasteurized chilled cream) of the purchased bulk pack was on its last day. There were many packs and we thought it unlikely that all the stock would be used in time. On top of which, the shelf life of the finished products produced that day containing the whipped cream would be up to 3 days after the manufacturer's use by date. The production manager disagreed that this was an issue as did the owner. I noted this as a major nonconformance in addition to a list of several minor nonconformances. The production inspection ended shortly after and as we walked to the bakery office to do the paperwork audit, my colleague turned around and saw the owner flipping us off.

As we reached the office, my colleague mentioned the owner's gesture. There was already a negative ambiance and discussing any point of improvement was a struggle. The quality manager was sidelined continually. The cream issue coupled with the management attitude gave me a bad feeling and led me to the decision to stop the audit and delist the supplier. Understandably the owner took umbrage, and our early departure was uncomfortable.

As per company procedure we immediately called our purchasing department to report the issue and discuss a way forward, who were in full support of the decision and launched the delist process. This also involved notifying the operational business that they could no longer order from this supplier. It was not an easy process as the operational business had an established relationship with the supplier. Changing supplier would be disruptive for them. But the head office procedure had been followed and the case closed.

Several weeks later we were contacted by our company's Environmental Health and Safety (EHS) team to report a serious food poisoning incident that had been linked to a big event where our company was catering. There were two suspected sources of contamination - one of which was the fresh cream patisserie dessert. It turned out that the operational business had continued to use the bakery supplier despite being instructed not to and having the central electronic payment system cut off.

It was never confirmed specifically which product or supplier caused the incident (whole genome sequencing did not exist then) but the operational business got a nasty shock and stopped using the supplier permanently.

Discussion and key learnings

- Food safety has been in jeopardy here because of the attitude of the supplier's owner - who did not take food safety management seriously - and of the management of the operational business - who felt that they could ignore an audit-driven delisting of one of their regular suppliers.
- Engaging operational colleagues as to why certain procedures are taken is essential. In this case the delist procedure was followed correctly (technical immediately informs the purchasing department who delists the supplier and informs the operation) but the decision

was not properly explained to the operation. They were informed to stop using the supplier, but the reason why was not fully explained. The delist action may have been seen as heavy-handed from the head office.

- An escalation process in the operation and aligning the leadership of different department streams would have been helpful in preventing the suppliers' continued use. For example, technical + buying + operation + EHS + finance.
- Fortunately, no one was seriously injured or died from the food poisoning. But it served as a lesson learnt for the operational business and was a helpful case study to illustrate why suppliers needed to be audited and that the technical services department existed to support the operational business (keep them out of trouble effectively).
- The paperwork was completed immediately with the list of nonconformances and details. This could be used as part of the incident investigation. The learning is to get the paperwork done right away!
- The coordination between different departments or groups is important to ensure proper implementation of decisions (Motarjemi, 2014).

References

Motarjemi, Y., 2014. Hazard analysis and critical control point (HACCP). Figure 31.2. In: Motarjemi, Y., Lelieveld, H. (Eds.), Food Safety Management-A Practical Guide for the Food Industry (Chapter 31). Academic Press, Waltham MA, pp. 845-872.

Further reading

GFSI, 2018. A Culture of Food Safety: A Position Paper from The Global Food Safety Initiative (GFSI). https://mygfsi.com/wp-content/uploads/2019/09/GFSI-Food-Safety-Culture- Full.pdf.

6.4 What to do when factories do not meet food safety standards?

It was a Friday and, as usual, at 10 a.m. we had our department management meeting. The members of the management team were the director and deputy director of the quality management department, the head of the food quality auditors, and myself, the corporate food safety manager of one of the leading multinational food companies. Incidentally, the head of the food quality auditors was absent that day.

As the only item on the agenda, the quality manager shared a document with great frustration and asked, "What should we do about this?" It was the report from the "corporate auditors," who worked under the direction of the Chief Financial Officer (CFO), as opposed to the food quality auditors. They had visited one of our facilities and rated the food safety situation at one of the plants as "unsatisfactory."

It should be noted that specific food quality and safety audits were also conducted as part of quality management, and those auditors reported directly to the director of quality management. One could argue that these audits lacked independence, a situation that was exacerbated by the authoritarian management style of the director of quality.

As the company's food safety manager, I was particularly concerned about the situation in the plant. On the one hand, I felt that allowing such a plant to continue to operate and market products would be inappropriate and a potential risk to public health. On the other hand, I knew that suggesting that the plant stop production would be seen as excessive by top management. Such a proposal would not be supported and, despite being the company's food safety manager, I simply did not have the authority to do so on my own initiative.

Rectifying this situation would anyway have serious financial implications and any recommendation I could make would still have to be approved by both the director of quality management and the director of operations. They both were primarily concerned with the bottom-line figures, and I did not expect much support.

So, I had to come up with a compromise solution. I suggested that we immediately send a team of experts to the plant to understand its problems in more detail and improve the situation.

To my astonishment, the director of quality management laughed at me and said, "No, this is not the way to handle such situations. Instead, we should call the plant manager and reprimand him for not being better prepared for the audit." Later, he sent a letter to all factories around the world, telling them that they should be well prepared for company audits.
Later, I recommended restructuring food safety management and creating an independent position responsible for food safety expert audits and whistleblowing situations. This position would report directly to the Chief Executive Officer (CEO). My proposal was rejected, and I was eventually terminated for my opinions. The company's management was then implicated in several incidents and later convicted in court for misconduct.

Discussion and learning points

This story raises several questions:

- Should corporate (financial) auditors be involved in food safety auditing?
- Is it appropriate to have food safety audits and internal grievance reporting (i.e., whistleblowing) as part of quality

assurance management system or should it be under an independent structure?

- What should be the responsibilities and authority of food safety managers?
- Should there be (separate?) systems of expert food safety audits? If so, where should they report?
- Should factories or production lines that do not meet a minimum food safety standard be allowed to produce and market products, or should they be shut down until the minimum requirements are met?

At present, regulatory authorities or international bodies have not taken a position on these questions. Regulatory authorities focus more on end products and incident management than on internal management principles and corporate compliance with internal policies. These issues need to be debated, decided, and developed further.

However, one thing is certain: plants must meet minimum food safety standards at all times, not just for audits.

Chapter Seven

Hygiene: risks and controls

7.1 Insects in pasta

I spent a week with a pasta factory in Europe. My task was to sign off on the corrective actions taken following a previous audit by a client and to prepare them for a later inspection. There had been several issues including ongoing customer complaints of insects in pasta. The producer had been temporarily delisted (by the client) and was keen to get reinstated. The factory was generally in good order, seemingly well run, and not visibly dirty. After a while, it became clear that there was tension between the Quality Assurance (QA) Manager and Production Director. The Managing Director kept himself out of the factory and focused on sales.

It took 2 days to go through the previous corrective actions - extra time was allocated to take into account the language differences and to prevent misunderstandings. The twice-daily wrap-up meetings with the management team and QA Manager were productive albeit long. Every point was vigorously discussed and sometimes arguments between the teams would break out. We still had no explanation for the insect contamination.

At the end of the second day's wrap up, the QA Manager complained that no one had been listening to his requests to deep clean the factory. An almighty argument broke out between him and the Production Director and after a highly emotional exchange, the QA Manager stormed out of the room in tears.

After an uncomfortable silence, I asked if we could start the next day before production so that I could get a better look at the incoming raw materials and production equipment before they were filled with product. The team agreed and early the next morning we entered the silent production hall with the QA Manager, the Production Director (PD), and the Managing Director (MD) accompanied by an engineer - on hand to dismantle equipment if needed.

I wove my way around the machinery (it would have been impossible to do this during production) and worked my way up a platform to one of the augers on the main production line that dispensed dough ready to be stamped and shaped. Leaning into the auger (again, not possible to do during production) I could see that sticking around the screw and in the crevices were old pieces of dough. We picked some of this off - many little insects were caked into it.

Indeed, the factory had not been subject to a deep clean for some time. Despite the QA Manager's requests, it took many customer complaints, suspended supply, an inspection, and finally taking the MD and PD into the factory for the QA Manager to be heard.

The insects were confused flour beetles (Tribolium confusum). We suspected that eggs which were trapped in the dough residue had hatched out over time. With a constant source of food and warmth, the insects had developed and multiplied, contaminating dough that was passing through the auger.
We also checked the incoming flour. The sieve checks were not being done effectively, leaving the potential for insects to enter. The barrel in which the sieve resided was opened and someone peered in once a week, but this did not allow the whole sieve area to be seen. The only way to properly check the sieve was intact and inspect contamination was to completely remove the sieve - a relatively simple action.

The MD instructed an immediate hold to production and to carry out a thorough deep clean. The cleaning schedule was updated and an employee was trained to operate the neglected steam cleaner.

Sieve checks were put into the regular maintenance schedule and any insects or visible eggs trapped in the sieve were reported to the flour supplier. The flour supplier was also scheduled for an audit.

Regular meetings with the QA Manager and management team were programmed to ensure feedback was properly actioned. The Human Resource (HR) Manager also became involved to provide support.

Discussion and key learnings

The events revealed that the PD was more concerned with producing as much volume in a given time than leaving time for proper cleaning and maintenance. He did not spend much time on the factory floor. The MD was hands off, leaving practical matters to the PD, who was also his brother. When the MD became aware for the reasons of the complaints and resulting delist, he resolved to pay more attention and ensure that his push for sales did not come at the cost of hygiene.

The additional time allocated early on to compensate for the language differences between myself and the QA Manager now had an extra benefit as the QA Manager relaxed enough over time to freely raise his concerns in front of his superiors. This meant we could get to the source of the issue quickly.

The breakdown in communication meant that relatively minor production issues became compounded over time and eventually led to lost business. The senior management attitude meant that complaints were not taken seriously and a thorough investigation of the root cause was not done.

An external party can be a helpful way to raise management awareness of problems. Although with the right internal management structure, processes, and food safety culture, this should not be needed.

Asking to see the factory floor before production starts can reveal hygiene issues that are impossible to see during full production. Conversely, of course, seeing the floor during production is needed to check the actual process and practices. Hygienic design of equipment is essential to prevent the accumulation of residues and allow effective cleaning.

Further reading

- A Culture of Food Safety, Global Food Safety Initiative, 2018. https://mygfsi.com/wp-   content/uploads/2019/09/GFSI-Food-Safety-Culture-Full.pdf.
- A-Z of Pests, British Pest Control Association. https://bpca.org. uk/a-z-of-pest-advice/flour-   beetle-control-how-to-get-rid-of-flour-beetles-bpca-pests/189153.
- Flour Beetles, Extension Entomology, Texas A&M Agrilife Extension Service. https:// extensionentomology.tamu.edu/ insects/flour-beetle/.
- Hygienic Design Principles, European Hygienic Engineering & Design Group (EHEDG). https://www.ehedg.org/guidelines/.

7.2 A foreign object is found in harvested product

"A client found hair in his spinach" were the words of a concerned catering manager reporting an incident that occurred in our operation. The complaint was recorded, batch details taken, supplier informed, and apology written to the client.

"A client found hair in her spinach" was reported again from the same operation, the complaints procedure followed, and this time the Environmental Health and Safety (EHS) team informed. It seemed that the catering unit was careless and probably not following the hair covering procedure.

Then, "A client found hair in his spinach" was reported for the third time, this time from another country but with the same supplier and batch of frozen spinach as the two previous complaints. The investigation now turned toward the supplier who was asked for remedial action.

"A client found hair in his spinach. We tested the hair and it really is hare - not rabbit," reported the EHS colleague from one country.

European-wide product recall of frozen spinach was instigated. The follow-up included a visit to the supplier, a large highly professional and competent producer. The investigation revealed that the spinach harvester had some missing front chains - these hang down and are there to shoo off small animals crouching among the crop. Unfortunately, a hare had passed through the gap in the chains and became entangled in the harvester, spreading itself out through the batch and into the factory. The washing and filtration systems were in good working order but the weight of the pieces of hare were light enough to pass through the entire system and end up in a block(s) of blanched frozen spinach.

Discussion and key learnings

- Assumptions were made that on hearing about "hair" in a meal that it was the kitchen staff not having protective covering. A description was not asked for nor given.
- If the piece of hare had not been tested and reported so quickly, we would likely have had many more complaints across many restaurants and countries.
- DNA testing at that time was not usual and it took some canny thinking from the EHS officer and laboratory to get it done.
- Growing and harvesting vegetables does not mean that animals do not get hurt in the process.

7.3 Glass in confectionery

It's 9 p.m. on a weeknight when Max the plant quality manager gets a call from the night quality supervisor at the plant. "Max, we have a problem" The second shift confections crew just opened one of the two in-line strainers on cook kettle number 2 and it's full of broken glass! Max immediately instructed her to shut down the operation and place all inventory of the product on embargo. "I will be driving in to the plant immediately." "It's going to be a long night."

Max has a lot to think about on his way to the plant. How did this happen? How much product is involved? Do we have it all? What needs to be done to prevent this in the future?

Background: The system feeding a single rotary filler makes a thick, sticky confectionery product that must be filled hot into glass jars. The filler runs at 80 jars per minute. If the filler stops for any reason, the product is diverted off into a drum lined with a heavy plastic bag. The product flow must continue or it will harden in the supply line. Drums were prelined (six deep) and open so that they could be put in place quickly if there was a line stoppage. The diverted product would then be taken back into the cook room and added to a cooker, melted, and pumped back into the main supply cooker. The melted product is run through one of 2¼ inch strainers that are parallel to each other. This is so the strainer could be switched at each shift, cleaned, and examined. The results would be manually recorded on a cook record sheet.

Investigation: The first step is to interview the second shift cook who found the problem. His story described how at the beginning of his shift he switched from using the left strainer to the right strainer. He then cleaned and examined the left strainer, reassembled it, and switched back to the left strainer. This was the same procedure done by the first and third shift cooks for at least 2 days. The cleaning would be done any time during the shift. The problem was that none of the cooks cleaned and examined the right strainer that was used while the left strainer was being cleaned. It contained several pieces of ground glass with the smaller pieces getting through the filter screen. Somehow a glass jar must have gotten into a fiber drum of product rework and got ground up by the pump that ran product through a strainer back into the main cook kettle. How did the glass get there? Recall the open barrels staged for a line shutdown. They were very near the filler, uncovered, and ready for diverted product. When there is a jar break in the filler or on the line, the procedure is to remove all open jars for 10 feet prior to and after the break. The filler operator would quickly throw the jars into open trash cans that were very close to the fiber barrels for divert product. The best theory ended up to be that a filler operator accidently threw one or more jars into a divert product drum instead of the trash can. Hence, the diverted product containing the jar(s) was added back and got ground up.

Discussion and key learnings

Statistical sampling designed by a professional statistician, aimed at detecting the onset of this problem, revealed a small number of affected jars from each shift for 2 days. Fortunately, all product was in control at the plant. The decision then was made to landfill all filled product from the 2 days and any filled drums of diverted product in inventory. The supervisor witnessing the product destruction described huge bulldozers crushing cases of product and diverted product drums with tracks covered in sticky product and broken glass. It was a scene not easily forgotten. The financial loss was sizable but fortunately the hazard was kept out of the market.

Design: Food production systems must always be designed to prevent entry of extraneous matter. In this case, the draw-off process was fundamentally flawed. The open drums next to a glass filler presented a hazard. The answer was to install a long, hot water jacketed line back to the cook kettle that would allow the diverted product to continuously flow. No more need for barrels. Initial production line design must involve quality/food safety professionals to ensure that product safety is always maintained and is built into the Hazard Analysis and Critical Control Points (HACCP) plan.

Training: The three shift cooks did not recognize that they were all cleaning the same strainer and not alternating as they were supposed to as per the HACCP plan. Refresher training was done so that they understood the need.

Quality assurance: Quality professionals must have proper check points to audit actual procedures and employee understanding of them. This should be formalized on a schedule and recorded.

7.4 Rodent droppings on fish

Auditing a small fish supplier, I felt a general unease. This was a first audit as the supplier had been listed following the acquisition of a food service operation. The owner was not open to improvements, and discussions were not constructive. As we entered the walk-in freezer, I had my boss's advice in my head, "When you are on your own during a visit, never walk into the freezer first."

Fortunately, the freezer inspection passed without incident to me, but the room was not well organized and there was no stock control.

We passed into the processing room which had been emptied for cleaning and was looking good on the surface, but I felt there was something strange. The owner was keen to speed me on, but I insisted on taking a deeper look. On a lower stainless steel table shelf were several packs of smoked salmon scattered with rodent droppings.

I ended the audit shortly after and the feedback discussion was difficult. The supplier had no intention of making improvements and had a blatant disregard for food safety.

Discussion and key learnings

- When visiting producers of unknown reputation, it makes sense to go accompanied.
- Follow your gut instinct and be wary of people who try to rush you through an area.
- Do not hesitate to end a visit that isn't going well.
- Over and above the negative attitude of the supplier, the mere fact that there were rodent droppings was

unacceptable. These are generally recognized as a serious source of food contamination.

Further reading

- BPCA (British Pest Control Association) Rattled by rats? Pest advice for controlling rats. https://bpca.org.uk/write/ MediaUploads/Documents/PestAware/BPCA_Rattled_by_ Rats_PestAware_Advice_Sheet.pdf.
- https://www.brcgs.com/media/638461/brc-bpg-pest-control-english-text.pdf. https://juniperpublishers.com/nfsij/pdf/NFSIJ. MS.ID.555683.pdf.
- GFSI. 2018. A Culture of Food Safety. A Position Paper from The Global Food Safety Initiative (GFSI). https://mygfsi.com/wp-content/uploads/2019/09/GFSI-Food-Safety-Culture- Full.pdf.

7.5 Ahmad's favorite laksa stall

It was a usual day when Ahmad bought his favorite laksa for his family from a local laksa stall. Laksa is a soup noodle popular in Southeast Asia. There are several types of laksa and the taste also can vary greatly by region. Two main noodle types used include thick wheat noodles and rice vermicelli. However, the broth can vary significantly ranging from spicy curry like broth to sour asam gelugur fish broth.

The laksa type in this story consists of thick wheat noodles, salad vegetables, egg, and sour asam gelugur soup. It is very popular not only to the local community but also to customers from other states, who will not miss the opportunity to buy and bring home packaged laksa. After Ahmad finished his work for the day, he stopped at the laksa stall that he frequented and bought several packages of laksa. His family had the laksa for dinner and not long after they began to experience symptoms such as fever, diarrhoea, and vomiting. They were admitted to a hospital, where it was suspected that they suffered from a food poisoning event. Sadly, it was not a minor food poisoning. After a few days in the hospital, one of the Ahmad's family members passed away from the illness.

Besides his family, there were also reports of consumers from other states who fell ill after consuming contaminated laksa from the same stall. Health officials conducted an investigation into the cause of the incident. Several food samples were taken and sent to the laboratory for analysis. The outbreak had claimed two lives and the culprit was later identified to be Salmonella which had contaminated the noodles. Poor hygiene conditions and handling practices at the laksa stall were thought to have caused the contamination and the outbreak.

Discussion and key learnings

Street foods have been very popular in many countries. They provide dietary variety at affordable prices and are popular to low-income and middle-income groups.

However, many vendors are known to operate under questionable hygienic conditions. Generally, many street food vendors lack refrigeration, clean water supply, and they prepare their foods in bulk earlier in the day. Additionally, cross contamination may also occur during the handling and preparation of food. In dangerous temperature zones, pathogens may grow.

Countries with a warmer climate and high consumption of street food run a higher risk of foodborne illness associated with street food. Furthermore, studies have shown that often, food safety knowledge of vendors is low and their attitude and practices are not optimal. These may further contribute to the poor hygienic quality of street food.

In some countries, all food operators must complete a food handler course before getting their license or permit, but this does not completely prevent cases of foodborne illness, because knowledge does not always lead to good behavior.
Thus, educating consumers on identifying food operators with good food handling practices will be crucial. Government departments responsible for food safety such as the department of health can play an important role in disseminating the information to the public through mass media, schools, and roadshows. Well- informed consumers will not purchase food from operators who compromise hygiene and safety. With increased demand from consumers for clean and hygienic street food, it will encourage the food operators to respect good hygienic practice.

An important learning point from this story is also that contrary to the general misperception that foodborne illnesses are benign and self-limiting, they can be deadly, particularly for those with poor health status. Generally, a low-income population is at greater risk.

Further reading

Motarjemi, Y., 2014. Public Health Measures: Health Education, Information and Risk Communication. Encyclopedia of Food Safety. Academic Press, Waltham, MA.

7.6 Recycling a mold problem

Working with a south-east Asian soy sauce producer, I was shown around the premises. A small group of ladies was working in a semi-open corner, washing bottles. The bottles - still full of product - were first emptied out in large garbage tons and collected in buckets. They were then put on a conveyor belt and transported to a machine with six filler heads, to be filled with - as it turned out -a sodium hypochlorite solution. A penetrating smell of bleach was in the air. Taking a closer look at the machine, it appeared that it was originally designed to first fill and then rotate and empty the bottles out, rotate them back, fill them with clean water, and rotate/empty them out again. But the machine would not rotate the bottles anymore, so the ladies took them off the conveyor belt, emptied them out by hand in a large vessel, sometimes up to their elbows in the bleach, and proceeded to rinse them out with water.

When I asked what this was all about, my hosts explained that they had previously washed the bottles on the machine with a detergent, rotated, and rinsed them out with water, but that had not been effective and they had been advised to change over to bleach. But that had corroded the machine, it didn't work anymore and the ladies had to do most of the cleaning by hand, without much protection. It still didn't do the job, they complained, and it also took too much space. And no, the ladies didn't complain about the work, they were happy to be employed. Was there anything that I could recommend to improve this situation?

Maybe I could, if they could first explain to me why we had all these dirty bottles on site in the first place. Those were product returns, they said, and cleaning those returned bottles was cheaper than buying new ones. But why so many, and why were they returned? It was mold, they said, and it was almost 40% of product shipped. Their brand was sold on the local markets only, so returns were collected together with the distribution of fresh product. When they found that the normal cleaning procedure would not do much to reduce the rate of mold infections and complaints, they had followed advice and replaced it with bleach.

My advice to them was to break the circle of recontamination: don't re-import bottles with molded product, don't mix them up with new bottles in the distribution chain, and don't wash dirty bottles on site. If bottles need to be washed out and disinfected, have that done separately in a place away from the factory, They should validate the effectiveness of the cleaning operation before allowing these bottles back on site. Also, please make sure that nobody has to get bleach on their hands and bare arms - and into their lungs.

What remained was the cleaning up of the rework area on the site, which would probably not be easy.

As the company was planning to move into an entirely new site anyway, it would be of the greatest importance to start operations there without recycling the mold problem.

Discussion and key learnings

Apart from the question how any company can stay in business if 40% of product is returned and needs to be destroyed (the owner had several businesses and had the expectation that this problem could be solved and he could expand the soy sauce business), this is good example of attempts to solve a problem without a root cause analysis. Bringing mold contamination back on site, dumping molded product into large open vessels, and reusing "cleaned" bottles, without any validation of the cleaning step, is asking for trouble. Changing over from normal industrial detergent to bleach is an attempt to address the effectiveness of a fundamentally flawed procedure again without any validation. In the process, a piece of equipment was destroyed (that spray cleaner will never work again) and, more importantly, workers' health was put at risk.

7.7 Hygiene issues in the food chain: finding the weakest link

The food production chain is often as strong as its weakest link. This is particularly true for fresh produce and products that must be delivered to the customers/consumers as clean as possible. Being involved in projects to assess and upgrade parts of the chain, my team became very much aware of the limitations of an isolated approach. One may be able to improve one step, only to be held back by other steps outside your control. Below are a few examples:

Bagged salad: A factory where fresh salads were processed and bagged to extend shelf life by improving hygiene. To hold bacteria count down, processing took place in a cooled environment, to a point that factory employees had to wear arctic parka coats, even during the summer. After inspecting all the processes, we took and analyzed a sample of the water transporting the vegetable leaves. We found a high count of fecal colonies in the water. As this water was continually recirculated, subsequent batches of vegetables were cross-contaminated. But where did the contamination come from? Many of the vegetables originated from Mediterranean countries. They arrived in bulk to be shredded and mixed at the factory. The farms where the produce originated used traditional organic fertilizer - the source of fecal coli bacteria. Additionally, no apparent effort had been made to ensure hygiene post-harvest.

For the factory, we could help to interrupt the recontamination loop by the contaminated water, but cleaning up the source of fecal coli upstream was another matter.

Refer containers: They are short for refrigerated containers that are used to transport fresh meat/meat products all over the world. Coming into Europe, EU legislation requires them to be washed down with a pressure hose. This practice may remove visible dirt, but forcefully spreads invisible contamination all around. After a visual inspection by veterinary authorities, they are released to be used again. We inspected one that was destined for Japan, with a load of pork. An Adenosine triphosphate (ATP) swab of the container predictably showed many areas of contamination. The air ducts from refrigeration units never get cleaned (the pressure hoses cannot get there), so any contaminants that can be carried by aerosols end up on the surfaces of the products that are transported. These containers are not ideally cleanable and hosing them down does not improve the situation much. What we need is a better hygienic design of the containers and legal requirements that make sense from a cleaning/sanitation point of view instead of "visually clean."

Pigsty hygiene: We examined hygiene at a large (5000 pigs/year) pig farming operation. Pigs are purchased at a local farm where they are bred. The farmer in this case study gets them when they are young. The farmer wanted to improve his operation and eliminate the use of antibiotics as much as possible. Improving general hygiene seemed to be the direction for a solution and we worked with a veterinarian to achieve that.

The farmer applied proper cleaning/disinfection techniques and we provided and instructed him with ATP swabs to check on status and progress. After a while he learned to get his stalls - between pig batches - to a level of cleanliness that would befit an average hospital ward. Then he and his team made an assay of the surfaces of the trucks that were bringing him new pigs and transporting the grown pigs to slaughter. The conclusion was these surfaces were not being cleaned properly even though the transporter, moving animals all across Europe, was certified for food safety. Going back further in the chain, it was found that the "nursery" where piglets are born also had inadequate cleaning and disinfection between old/new groups of animals.

A chicken slaughter facility had made an application to expand its production. It would add jobs in the area, but local authorities would not give permission. There were already problems with excessive volume and organic load of the effluents from the plant. The local water treatment plant was overwhelmed by the high levels of coli bacteria. When we got involved, the level of coli in the samples was many times higher than what would be acceptable, and it impacted the beach and the safety of swimming water.

At the office of the water treatment plant, we learned that a bank of ultraviolet (UV) lights had been installed to kill the bacteria but that did not work - the water was too murky for the light to penetrate effectively. Also, a filtration system was installed but that did not solve the problem either. A new, experimental, technology seemed to be able to reduce the coli count to less than one. It would cost a fraction of the UV and filter applications, but the water treatment plant did not dare to go back to the city council and ask for more money, having to explain that what had already been spent did not work.

Discussion and key learnings

All four cases demonstrate that food (or water) safety critically depends on the basics of hygienic design - across the entire food chain. That includes cleanability (the ducts in the containers), the prevention of contamination (the salad from the organically fertilized farms), the actual cleaning (pigsty and transport), and the basic willingness to admit past failures (which may have been made in perfectly good faith) and move on to something that works (the chicken/water treatment). Food and water safety requires an integrated approach, though we may only get there step by step, with all the imperfections and disappointments along the way. The recent emphasis on "food safety culture" seems to recognize this and might help to address instances as described earlier.

7.8 A dangerous past

A toxicologist once said to me - somewhat sarcastically - that he did not know of any substance that had not become 10 times more toxic in the last 10 years. That may sound a bit strange, but it actually does reflect our increasing understanding of the dangers of substances that were freely used in the past, but were only recently investigated for their health effects.

Some of those chemicals ended up being simply dumped into the environment, only to raise their ugly heads later, unexpectedly, and with very negative consequences.

A few weeks ago, I learned about a family who had been tested for extremely high levels of PFOS (perfluorooctanesulfonic acid) in their bodies. The news article went on to say that the substance was found in ecological beef from a local farmer, implicitly (but erroneously) suggesting that eating organic beef could be harmful to the health. On further investigation, we came to the conclusion that PFOS - once used in surface treatment and fire retardants - had ended up on the pastures of the ecological farm. The farmer never suspected that he unwittingly poisoned his cattle and his customers.

In a separate case, a multinational company which recycles newspaper had come to us looking for solution to hydrogen sulfide (H2S) dangers in their production factory. Two employees had died from exposure to the gas. The company had several plants globally. An initial check at one plant showed that the wastewater from production was poured into a 15-meter deep, 15-meter diameter settling tank to reduce the overall volume, for which they would otherwise be charged a fee as wastewater. The settling tank was periodically emptied, and the cellulose waste given to a local farmer who spread it on his ground. PAHs (polyaromatic hydrocarbons) had been discovered in the water but the city wastewater engineer had cooperated with a local beef slaughterhouse to dilute their combined effluent to below acceptable limits. Examination of the processes in the factory showed that the PAHs came from the place where deinking took place, whereas H2S is a problem for many sewage lines where there is decaying organic material. If they had addressed the problem at the source, as legislation requires, the whole problem would have been solved. Instead, workers were exposed to toxic H2S gas, wastewater contained PAHs, and farmland was probably contaminated. To our knowledge, no analysis has ever been made of the accumulation of PAHs in the production from the farm whether for animal or human consumption.

Discussion and key learnings

Regarding the chemicals involved, PFOS and related compounds like per- and polyfluoroalkyl substances (PFAS) (various surface treatment chemicals) and other persistent organic pollutants are now banned for production in Europe. They are included in the category of organic pollutants that accumulate in the food chain and are covered by the "Stockholm Convention." The two stories illustrate the need for "chemical archeological" investigations along the food chain. Harmful substances may have been applied or dumped in places where they persist and will do harm, possibly unnoticed for many years. A lot of these problems could have been prevented, but not all authorities and institutions involved have the motivation or the resources to start digging for problems. Still, national databases for authorities with jurisdiction on environmental protection could be a place to start looking for signs and eventual prevention.

Recent news about pollution levels of soil and water wells seems to underline both the scope and the seriousness of the issue, which will require very major effort and will be with us for the foreseeable future.

Professor Philippe Grandjean, the head of the Environmental Medicine Research Unit at the University of Southern Denmark, stated recently that the problem of these substances will take decades to solve. "145 areas are being investigated for toxic substances but this is only the top of the iceberg."

Further reading

- EEA (European Environment Agency). 2021. Emerging chemical risks in Europe "PFAS". https://www.eea.europa.eu/publications/emerging-chemical-risks-in-europe.
- Jydskevestkysten.2021.145 område derundersøgesforgiftstof:Mendet er kun toppen af isb- jerget, advarer professor. https://kobenhavnliv.dk/artikel/145-omr%C3%A5der-unders%C3%B8ges-for-giftstof-men-det-er-kun-toppen-af-isbjerget-advarer-professor.
- EWG (The Environmental Working Group). 2021. Mapping the PFAS contamination crisis: New data show 2,854 sites in 50 states and two territories. https://www.ewg.org/ interactive-maps/pfas_contamination/. (USA).
- Stockholm Convention. www.pops.int.
- Denmark News in English. https://www2.mst.dk/udgiv/publications/2015/04/978-87-93283- 01-5.pdf.
- What are PFAS and how are they dangerous for my health? www.eea.europa.eu/help/faq/ what-are-pfas-and-how. https://www.eea.europa.eu/data-and-maps/indicators/hazardous-substances-in-marine-organisms-3/assessment.

7.9 Foreign material prevention gone wrong

Visiting a plant to do an inspection, I looked into a kettle with a flashlight and saw an accumulation of material, whereas the kettle was supposed to be clean at that point. As it turned out, the material consisted of clams - an allergen. For some reason, the cleaning clearly had not been effective and as a result product might now be contaminated and have to be recalled. Maintenance explained that they had welded a cross made of stainless-steel bar resembling an X over the three-inch discharge pipe leading out of the kettle. But why would they do that, especially now that this crossbar was collecting allergenic residue material? It was to protect the product from being contaminated with foreign materials, I was told. And they explained to me what had happened.

This stainless-steel cooking kettle, used for mixing and heating for dairy products such as dips with ingredients such as peppers, spices, and flavorings, had a constantly rotating scraper to ensure thorough mixing and to avoid burning of material on the heated product contact surface. Burn on material had to be removed prior to running the next batch of product. That is normal practice.

The scraping was done with a flexible material, but at the cleaning process (after each batch), aggressive chemicals at elevated temperature were (and typically are) used to remove the burnt-on material. These chemicals overtime degrade the scraper material and cause it to be brittle and easily fractured or broken.

The plant had no program to replace the scrapers periodically, so they would gradually shatter and cause foreign material contamination. The broken pieces would fall into the liquid and be passed through the pump which propels the product to the next processing step or to the packaging fillers. This had resulted in plastic pieces getting into the product stream and in the final package.

The maintenance team had a solution! They would stop broken scraper blades from entering the discharge pipe and being pulled into the pump and broken into small pieces by welding this stainless-steel crossbar in front of the discharge pipe, which I had seen (beneath the clams). The maintenance team ensured that the welds were polished and they looked sanitary to them.

They had also considered to replace the scraper blades on a periodic basis and thereby prevent the breakage issue altogether, but decided against that. The cost per scraper was less than $40 per blade, with the number of blades depending on the size of the kettle (they had a number of these kettles, various sizes). Maintenance and Quality Assurance (QA) felt comfortable with the chosen solution, it was helpful in reducing plastic-related consumer complaints.

But then a new product was introduced using the scraped surface kettle, which contained an allergen - mollusks. The specific product was a clam-based dip with long stringy clams added -and now suddenly we had a serious food safety issued cross-contamination from an allergen.

As a result, the plant recalled subsequent production since it was exposed and likely contained some of the clams from the crossbar, at a total cost in the area of $300,000.

Discussion and key learnings

- Running equipment beyond its breaking point and then filtering out the pieces is never a good idea and the introduction of an allergen-containing product variation then precipitated a crisis that could have been prevented.
- A preferred approach would be to establish a preventive maintenance task to inspect the blades on a frequent basis (e.g., weekly, of after a fixed number of production/cleaning cycles) and then change the blades at a set frequency before material deterioration and breakage would set in.
- The introduction of a new product - especially one with an allergenic ingredient - requires a reconsideration of the risk assessment around the process. This especially involves the cleaning process, cross-contamination, and the prevention of accumulation of residual material.
- With any change, there is the question: "what will cause the change to fail?" Will changes be safe for new product introductions? Critical thinking is needed to explore all possibilities.

7.10 Failures in incident investigation and root cause analysis

One day we learned that in a Latin American country, a few hundred dogs had died from poisoning with our pet food products. It was contaminated with a high level of aflatoxin.

An investigation into the incident showed that the factory where the pet food was produced had transferred the responsibility for testing the raw material, maize, to the supplier. The supplier carried out its tests on samples taken from batches of maize that were different from the moldy and poor-quality maize it supplied to our plant.

At the time, our pet food business was considered a separate business and had its own technical management. I was told that I was not responsible for this business and that I had no right to interfere in its management. Nor did I have a job description defining the limits of my responsibilities.

However, when this incident occurred, I suddenly became accountable for the incident. Top management asked me to explain what instructions I had given to the plant. Fortunately, together with the technical management of the pet food company and my team, I had issued an instruction that all raw materials had to be checked and tested for aflatoxin content. We also prescribed control measures all along the production process, including a final test and verification of the finished product.

As per our instruction, our factory tested the final product, but the test results showing a much higher level of contamination than the raw material were not reviewed and were not compared to the negative test results provided by the supplier. An audit of the factory by one of my colleagues in the department had not detected the problem either.

To the good fortune of the company, the incident did not make much of a stir in the media. This was because at the same time as this event, a major landslide made many victims and caused a lot of damage.

Management concluded that I had in no way failed in my responsibilities as I had given the correct instructions. The plant's quality manager was immediately dismissed, even before an investigation into the root cause of the problem could be conducted. And so, we never had answers to the relevant questions in this case: Who had decided that the raw material tests should be delegated to the supplier? Why did the supplier commit such fraud and how was it possible that the factory remained unaware of the poor quality of the maize? Were they aware of the dogs' vulnerability to aflatoxin? Why were the results of the finished products not checked and followed up? Why didn't the auditor detect the problem? No answers, no further investigation, it almost looked like a cover-up.

Curiously, in all the years I worked at the company's headquarters, the regulatory authorities never investigated management's role in the incidents. Not even when there was a fatal incident. Also, lessons from our incidents and crisis were never published internationally to benefit the food supply and improve the foundations of the food safety management systems.

Discussion and key learnings

Domestic animals are particularly sensitive to aflatoxins, and control measures, such as testing a raw material that may present such a risk, are critical. The factory in question had made a major mistake in delegating the responsibility for testing the raw material to this supplier. While asking suppliers for a certificate of analysis on incoming materials is not uncommon, the testing is supposed to be carried out on samples of the actual shipped batch and not on unrelated "golden samples." This practice is a clear sign of bad faith and an indication that the supplier knew that the materials delivered were contaminated.

The whole situation would still have been discovered at an early stage, if somebody would have checked the results of the tests carried out on the finished product, but they did not, which is at least a serious dereliction of duty, but not entirely uncommon, especially when staff are overwhelmed, or departments work in silos.

In this case, the superficial investigation after the incident and the failure to analyze the root causes of the incident was also a significant error. It was wrong to dismiss the plant's quality manager before the incident was thoroughly investigated and responsibilities established, also because a key witness now could no longer be interviewed.

We are again reminded that audits cannot detect all problems and it is only the competence and ethics of personnel which can be the guarantee for safety.

Finally, responsibilities and accountabilities were not clear in the company. This is a major problem in terms of food safety management.

From a regulatory perspective, incidents are rarely investigated up to management level, to determine roles and responsibilities and hold people accountable. Often the quality manager is considered the culprit and dismissed, sometimes even before a full investigation is carried out. This undermines the possibility of a full investigation.

Analyzing the root causes of incidents and publishing the lessons learned would be a valuable tool for other companies to learn and improve their systems and practices.

Further reading

- Carrion, P.A., Thompson, L.J., 2014. Pet food. Chapter 15. In: Motarjemi, Y., Lelieveld, H. (Eds.), Food Safety Management: A Practical Guide for the Food Industry. Academic Press, Waltham MA ,pp. 379- 396.
- Motarjemi, Y., 2014. Hazard analysis and critical control point system (HACCP). In: Motarjemi, Y., Lelieveld, H. (Eds.), Food Safety Management : A Practical Guide for the Food Industry. Academic Press, Waltham MA ,pp. 845-872.
- Motarjemi, Y., Wallace, C., 2014. In: Motarjemi, Y., Lelieveld, H. (Eds.), Incident and Root Cause Analysis in Food Safety Management : A Practical Guide for the Food Industry. Academic Press, Waltham MA, pp. 1017-1036.

7.11 And it burns, burns, burns

A few years ago, the management of a company producing cakes containing fillings with a high microbiological sensitivity, such as fresh whipped cream, soft cheese, or other dairy spreads, asked me to explain what went wrong with their products, because they did not meet the microbiological criteria set for this type of products. The management claimed that good hygiene practices (GHP), good manufacturing practices (GMP), and a food safety system (Hazard Analysis Critical Control Points [HACCP]) were implemented, but products still tested unsatisfactory when assessed against the official food safety criteria.

After sampling the processing environment and ingredients, I was prepared to take samples from the hands of food-handling workers when I noticed that their palms had very dry and chapped skin. Asking the food handlers about the procedure they used to wash and disinfect their hands, they confessed they are not very much inclined to apply it as they were trying to avoid the disinfection phase, because it involved a solution of sodium hypochlorite, which damaged their skin. So, the food handlers washed and disinfected their hands only when a supervisor was around.

Based on this finding, I recommended to the company managers to change the disinfectant to one based on alcohol. After this intervention, the workers started to wash and disinfect their hands as many times as necessary and the products started to comply with microbiological criteria.

Discussion and key learnings

As a substantial proportion of foodborne outbreaks are caused by food contaminated by food workers, personal hygiene is an important part of GHP. Washing hands with soap and warm water for 20 s before handling food is necessary because our hands become contaminated with microorganisms and act as vehicles to transfer them to food. Hands need to be washed very often (before starting work, after using the restrooms, after eating, drinking, using tobacco, after coughing, sneezing, or using a tissue or a handkerchief, before putting on gloves, after touching raw ingredients or surfaces touched by them, after touching garbage, handling dirty equipment or utensils, and after touching the body). Washing hands using regular soap and warm water and applying a proper hand washing technique will be enough to ensure hands are clean, but disinfection assures that potentially remaining pathogens are killed. Wash hands then disinfect them as, otherwise, these chemicals will be much less effective.

Disinfectants should be utilized in line with their usage guidelines. While chlorine-based disinfectants are inexpensive (the reason for which the managers from the cake company chose one of them) and have relatively quick kill times, they are corrosive, cause discoloration and irritation, so they do not have to be used on metals and on skin. Instead, alcohols, quaternary ammonium compounds (quats), and hydrogen peroxide are dermatologically compatible. When setting hygiene procedures, food safety managers have to ensure themselves that procedures are feasible and do not harm the workers. In case of noncompliance, it is important to understand the reason for it.

A table for comparison of disinfectants for surfaces in the food industry allows to choose a disinfectant based on its properties. (Sanosil). Do not forget that "good hygiene doesn't cost, it pays!"

Reference

Sanosil. What are surface disinfectant products? https://www.
sanosil.com/en/product-lines/ surface-disinfection/.

Further reading

- https://www.manorlaborator.ro/assets/legislatie/Ordin%20%20
  27%20_2011%20.pdf.
- https://www.sanosil.com/en/product-lines/surface-disinfection/

7.12 Foodborne intoxication caused by eating street food

In January 2019, an intoxication implicating street food caught my attention. The Food Safety Management Board in my country announced that 88 people had been hospitalized for emergency treatment for foodborne illness, with symptoms of vomiting and diarrhoea, at a local hospital. An investigation team was put together.

The patients declared that they had eaten bread with a filling of cold meat, rolls, egg sauce, pate, ham, pickles, and raw vegetables, all bought at one particular bread trolley. The team took samples of the mentioned ingredients for testing. The results showed that, in violation of regulatory standards, samples of ham and raw vegetables were contaminated with Salmonella, while pickles were contaminated with Clostridium perfringens.

The remaining food at this stall was destroyed in accordance with government regulations.

The owner of bread trolley that caused the outbreak was fined for violating various hygiene regulations, including not separating raw materials and (semi) finished products and not separating processing and non-food areas, leading to foodborne infections. Despite the high number of victims, the transgressions were not seen as sufficiently serious to be prosecuted for criminal liability. In addition to fines, the vendor was prohibited from selling bread with mixed ingredients for 4 months.

Discussion and key learnings

Street food items, being nutritious and low cost, available in easy-to-reach locations, are commonly found in our country.

This artisanal food industry feeds millions of people every day and employs millions of skilled and unskilled sellers, earning billions of dollars in income. However, it presents its own challenges in terms of food safety, hygiene, and the environment.

According to statistics of the Food Safety Department of the Ministry of Health, there are more than 1000 cases of foodborne illness per year. Street food contaminated with pathogens accounts for a great proportion of cases - investigations have shown that approximately 80% of vendors' hands selling food on sidewalks were contaminated with E. coli bacteria.

The present story is an example of outbreaks related to street food. Although the investigation was not complete in terms of identifying the nature of illness of the patients, the link between contamination and the practice of street food vendors (for instance, time-temperature abuse) would have been a possible cause of intoxication with C. perfringens; it did provide evidence of contamination of street foods.

In view of the cultural importance of street food, education and training of street food need to be reinforced at the same time that consumers need to be made aware to recognize high-risk products and unsanitary conditions of street food preparation.

Further reading

The following references are originally in Vietnamese. Online translation available.

- https://vfa.gov.vn/chi-dao-dieu-hanh/kiem-soat-ngo-doc-thuc-pham-thuc-an-duong-pho.html.

- https://phongkhambinhminh.com.vn/moi-truong-songgiam-nguy-co-ngo-doc-thuc-pham-tu-thuc-an-duong-pho.html.
- https://trungtamytephuxuyen.vn/index.php/bai-tuyen-truyen/bai-tuyen-truyen-thuc-an-duong- pho-128.html.

7.13 Pesticide poisoning in agriculture

The dependency of farming on toxic chemicals is a major concern. Too many chemicals used in the fields and gardens will affect farmers' health as well as consumers of agricultural products.

Despite efforts to reduce the use of toxic chemicals in agriculture, the use of pesticides and herbicides is still widespread in some South-East Asian countries and it has negative effects on farmers' health, food safety, and living environment. The excessive use of pesticides leads to high levels of pesticide residues in agricultural products, soil, water, and air environment.

Personally, I have seen that farmers often do not pay much attention to the toxicity warning symbols on the package and do not understand the dangers of pesticides. In most cases it appears that they are primarily interested in the effectiveness of the pesticides for crops and financial considerations. In many cases farmers prefer to use a higher dose of pesticides than recommended on the label, expecting increased effectiveness.

In 2019, we conducted a survey with 300 households in three communities. Results indicated that 99% of the surveyed farmers used pesticides, but only 10% of them used the pesticides as recommended by professional organizations, 92% used sprays based on their own experience in the control of pests in their crops, and 27% frequently sprayed even when there were no pests. Similarly, 95% of the farmers surveyed used herbicides in their crops, of which only 4% used it as recommended, 88% sprayed when weeds were present, and 39% regularly sprayed even when there was little grass.

Discussion and key learnings

The observations made earlier are corroborated with other studies. At the end of 2018, a test result from the Institute of Environmental and Occupational Health in my country showed that 31 out of 67 people that had been tested in four suburban districts had pesticide residues in their blood. According to the report, from 2017 to May 2019, 462 poisoning cases were associated with pesticides in only one province. In particular, poisoning caused by drinking water containing herbicides in 2018 led to 78 people being hospitalized. Many people in this group were employees, officials living in communities and towns without a direct relation to agricultural production. It can be inferred that with a large number of pesticides that are used indiscriminately today, many of which that are of unknown origin have a significant impact on public health.

All pesticides have negative effects on human health if used at too high levels and through inappropriate procedures, for example, applying pesticides without wearing gloves and protective gear, or though inhalation. Pesticides may also find their way into the human body through the food chain, especially fruits and vegetables.

People need to be (made) aware of the risks involved and, in my country, (and many others) we need clear legislation and a continuous campaign to educate farmers and consumers about (selective, targeted) pesticides. For instance: how pesticides should be labeled, the proper ways to apply them (personal protection, amounts of pesticide to be used, appropriate weather conditions), and when to harvest products after application. Consumers must routinely wash or peel products to minimize their intake of pesticides.

Further reading

The following references are originally in Vietnamese. Online translation available.

- https://bvndtp.org.vn/ngo-doc-thuoc-bao-ve-thuc-vat/. https://www.chongdoc.org.vn/cap-cuu-ngo-doc-cac-hoa-chat-bao-ve-thuc-vat-29336.
- https://moh.gov.vn/web/phong-chong-benh-nghe-nghiep/thong-tin-hoat-dong/-/asset_publisher/content/dieu-duong-cham-soc-benh-nhan-ngo-doc-thuoc-tru-sau.

7.14 A better mouse trap: integrated pest management

Early in my career, I had the fortunate opportunities to travel to many countries, experience wonderful cultures, and to practice my rudimentary language skills in Spanish. I was very excited at my first opportunity to visit a Biscuit Manufacturing company in Central America. The company was typical of a Biscuit company with an integrated system from flour receiving and sifting, to mixing of dry materials with water and oil, and to the molding of the dough into various shapes for baking and packaging. The food safety control measures were also typical, with high temperatures for baking for biological hazards, use of magnets and metal detection systems for foreign bodies, and with the final product intrinsic properties of low moisture/low water activity to ensure safety and stability.

I started my facility inspection in the morning at the dry goods warehouse, accompanied by a Quality Manager, who also was my translator. Pallets of material were stacked from floor to ceiling, close to the walls, and not readily accessible for inspection. Rodent glue boards were placed at various intervals, and all covered with flour dust. I explained to the Quality Manger that the glue boards would probably not be effective in this environment, particularly one in which the housekeeping was hard to maintain. I describe how a rodent bait station could be more effective. The Quality Manager quickly explained "La Ratta Grande" that what they have was too big to fit in a bait station and that "Jose" was more effective. It turned out that "Jose" was the first person on the morning shift and he used a club. However, La Ratta usually comes back.

Discussion and key learnings

The Biscuit Manufacturing company had an ineffective pest management program. Pallets stacked closed to walls made it difficult to execute inspection-monitoring as well as providing a harbourage site for pest. Poor housekeeping means potentially available food for insects, rodents, and other pests. Rodent glue boards were not effective in a dusty environment (and are no longer allowed in some countries as being unnecessarily cruel). "La Ratta Grande" coming back indicates probable entry into the facility that has become "home."

This situation exemplifies traditional pest management that relies on monitoring and reacting to visual evidence of pest with controls such as insecticides, rodenticides, use of traps, and in this case "Jose." These controls ultimately may be ineffective without the understanding of the biological and physical nature of the pest and to leverage their vulnerability for control, which is the foundation of the Integrated Pest Management (IPM) approach. IPM can be described an action-oriented process that uses the most appropriate pest control methods and strategies in an environmentally and economically sound manner to meet a desired pest management objective.

Key elements of an effective IPM program include (1) inspection and documentation of external and internal facility vulnerable areas, (2) defining an action threshold to trigger when control must be taken, (3) execution and evaluation of the effectiveness of control, and (4) education of personnel - particularly on the nature of the pest and of appropriate controls to be used. Prerequisite to establishing an IPM program should be fundamental knowledge of the identified pest and with priorities on eliminating potential sources of food, water, and shelter. Eliminating potential facility entry points and maintaining good housekeeping and cleaning/sanitation programs are essential in controlling food, water, and potential pest shelter and breeding area.

Further reading

Vastano, B., Chaven, S. (Eds.), June 1, 2009. IPM: a practical approach to pest control. Food Safety Magazine. https://www.food-safety.com/articles/3913-ipm-a-practicalapproach-to-pest-control.

7.15 "Mankoushe": gluten exposure

The bakery where I usually order my morning treats gave us a scare and it was no Halloween trick. It started soon after a customer, who we shall call James, walked into the bakery and explained to the owner that he is allergic to gluten and that he has brought his own corn bread, gluten-free dough loaves that he would like to have baked into "Mankoushe" - a traditional, famous Levantine food, similar to pizza, but made solely with thyme mixed with olive oil, placed on the flat dough. The baker reassured James and asked him to return to collect them in an hour.

So, James returned, collected his fresh, hot mouth-watering "Mankoushe," and headed back home for his breakfast. Soon after, I saw an ambulance rush past the bakery where some friends and I were having our breakfast. When we asked what the issue was, we learned that it was James having a strong allergic reaction that required immediate medical attention. The baker was puzzled and started to explain himself that he only used the dough that James had given him. However, when I investigated more, I understood that the baker was not fully aware about the possibility of cross-contamination and he was not careful while handling James's food as it was placed on the same tile which had gluten flour on. Moreover, the baker handled the dough without changing gloves while his hands were covered with flour from a previous mix. Also, he used a roller that was used to roll other products. James was thankfully treated quickly - although he manifested hard swollen bumps with severe skin rash all over his body - and did not pursue legal action against the baker, who was an old man.

Discussion and key learnings

Seven main food safety principles had been ignored in this case:

1. a consumer with a known allergy using a place where allergens were not adequately managed;

2. proper safety measures such as washing hands and cleaning surfaces between different dishes with and without certain allergens were not implemented;

3. utensils were not cleaned before each usage, especially when used to prepare meals containing allergens,

4. there was no awareness and proper communication among staff members when an order came in from an allergic customer;

5. a clear process should have been in place to ensure that the food can be safely prepared and served to the correct customer;

6. segregation of tools and space should have been available in order to facilitate division of labor; and

7. the baker should have been more aware of the risks associated with allergens and should not have accepted this order knowing that the end product would be contaminated with residues from the workplace.

Further reading

Wen, H., Kwon, J., 2016. Food Protec. Trends. 36 (5), 72-383.

7.16 Travel-related foodborne illness: salad versus chicken

In my life, I have traveled extensively to countries with low levels of hygiene. Once, with a small group of fellow friends, we were on an organized trip, visiting mysterious and culturally rich countries. We were particularly careful and attentive to hygienc. Because of my expertise, I took responsibility for the food safety aspects and warned about food hygiene issues, such as not taking ice in our drinks or eating suspect street food. We took as much care as possible.

We were on our way back from Syria, a culturally and historically amazing country, with a four-wheeled car, when we decided to make the last stop just before the border of Turkey. We were exhausted and hungry, we wanted to eat something. There was only one restaurant, and we were eager to order something to eat. There were two choices: green salad and fried chicken. Of course, everyone wanted to have something green after all, but we restricted ourselves, not to eat something raw, especially no raw salad. So, for dinner we had to sacrifice some chicken. However, against our very clear recommendation, one of our team members ordered a raw salad. Ironically, we started joking about the use of our remaining activated charcoal tablets at the end of the trip. We had barely crossed the Syrian-Turkish border when the travel companion who had eaten a salad began to experience symptoms of illness (vomiting, red spots), but nothing typical of the more well-known foodborne illnesses. So, we stopped near the border at a well-equipped Turkish hospital. There, a viral infection was suspected. After a few hours of treatment, our colleague was discharged. Later, she admitted to seeing the cook, working in an open-air kitchen, licking the fork he was using to mix the salad. Did he contaminate the salad, or was the salad contaminated from another source? We will never know because there was no investigation into the source of infection.

We were just glad to be back in our country, as we knew the story could have ended with a much worse outcome.

Discussion and key learnings

The story highlights the fact that food safety is an important issue for travelers and that they need to be aware of potential risks and what foods are safe to eat. In addition, it underscores the importance of reporting and investigation. In principle, food inspection services should be alerted to check the restaurant, investigate the possible source of the contamination, and, if necessary, take corrective action.

Chapter Eight

Food fraud and counterfeiting

8.1 Beef, the deceptions

Growing up in a little village in Africa, it was a privilege to be served a meal with beef from the local slaughterhouse. The car tire smoked beef had a sweet, roasted aroma when used in soups and stews preparation. Car tires were used to burn or singe the furs off the skin of the cattle slaughtered for sale to the public. Little did we know of the range of carcinogenic, teratogenic, and mutagenic chemicals formed and released by the process and the associated effects to humans and the environment. Officials from the veterinary office of the Local Assembly and some other concerned organizations began education on the environmental and health implications of these practices in meat processing and have since issued a ban on the use of car tire burning in meat processing. The education exercise which involved both the butchers and the general public had some positive impact on meat processing in our country. Some slaughterhouses changed over to alternative sources of heat (like gas) for the meat singeing, and most households, including mine, also began buying beef from safe slaughterhouses and cold stores which had started springing up in the communities. The new emerging cold stores mainly sold imported meat and meat products.

However, the purchase of beef from cold stores also came with a different challenge. One fateful Saturday in the year 2011, I bought beef from a cold store in the market to use in preparing stew for my family. In the process of peeling the wrapper from the beef, I decided to read the label (which I usually do not do). It said that this was buffalo meat. Not sure what buffalo meat was, I asked my husband, "Dear, what is buffalo?" And he said "buffalo referred to a male cow." Satisfied with his answer, I went ahead and used the meat to prepare a meal for my family which we really enjoyed. Days passed by and the word buffalo kept ringing in my head, so I decided to verify. To my surprise, buffalo was a different bovine species. And so, the next time I went to buy beef from the cold store, I emphatically asked the shop attendant to give me "original" beef. He responded, "Madam if you want cow meat, buy from the slaughterhouse. All cold stores in the market sell buffalo meat as beef." Short of words, I left the store.

Discussion and key learnings

- Drying or singeing food in any form over open fire of any kind is problematic because of the formation of toxic chemicals. Burning car tires takes this problem to an extreme.
- Selling "beef" that really is from a different species - usually for price/profit reasons - has happened in other places too. And it is not just beef - every high value product is at risk from being copied, faked, counterfeited (fish, olive oil, clothing, watches, etc.).
- In this case the labels faithfully mentioned the type of meat, but that still won't matter unless consumers actually read the label.
- Even the best husbands don't know everything.

Further reading

Wilson, W.G., 2005. Wilson's Practical Meat Inspection, seventh ed. Blackwell Publishing, pp. 8-83. 229-231.

8.2 Economic adulteration of ingredients with unapproved food colorants

In the early 2000s, Europe experienced a series of incidents related to non-food approved colorants. The first major incident occurred in the United Kingdom and affected both branded and own label products in various food sectors. The culprit was paprika adulterated with Sudan I (red), a dye that is commonly used in homecare products. The colorant was in an ingredient used in a well-known brand of Worcester sauce, which in turn had been used as a flavoring ingredient in other formulated products, ranging from crisps, dehydrated noodle snacks, soups, sauces, and frozen and chilled entrees. Given the usage of Worcester sauce within the finished products was low and the level of paprika used as an ingredient in the Worcester sauce was low, the level of Sudan 1 in the finished products was either at or between the limit of quantitation and the limits of detection for the analytical methods used at that time.

The contamination of Sudan 1 had been identified by the manufacturer of the Worcester sauce within the paprika, which originated from India. The UK's Food Standards Agency (FSA) had been informed and they demanded the names of all companies that had been supplied with the contaminated sauce.

Our company was informed by both the vendor and the FSA. The FSA's rationale and demands were very simple; the colorant was not approved for food use and irrespective of the level in the finished product even if not detectable it was identified as present through traceability. Therefore, it must be removed from sale. The FSA also published the findings on their website and named all brands and own label products impacted. Chaos ensued, with coverage of brands on shelf on all news bulletins throughout the day and evening for several days of that week. The impact across the United Kingdom was enormous increasing pressure on retailers and manufacturers to publicly recall products from the market. Damage to affected brands was enormous, with lost sales of 25%-30%) in several cases further compounded over the subsequent months. In several cases, the level of Sudan 1 in the product was parts per 100 trillion range. Nevertheless, the FSA insisted on action, which was complied with and damaged brand reputations and sales into the future. This type of contamination is still an issue to the present day.

Discussion and key learnings

The Sudan red incident caught the food industry by surprise, and one might say off guard. Adulteration of food materials with non-food ingredients has a long history and they present a particular problem for the food industry, because it is difficult to analyze raw materials if you don't know what you are looking for. Avoiding traders - who typically buy from uncontrolled sources - and requiring internationally recognized certification and traceability assurances from vendors are helpful precautions. Where analyses are carried out, it is critically important to use certified laboratories and accredited methods. Food companies are also well advised to actively monitor relevant news sources (including consumer organizations and nongovernmental organization (NGOs), who regularly carry out and publish analyses, but don't always inform the brand owners directly) for any signs of emerging issues.

8.3 Horse gate: the European meat adulteration scandal

In Ireland, December 2012, the Irish Foods Standards Agency (FSAI) carried routine compositional surveillance on a range of beef containing frozen foods. One of the analytical techniques employed was polymerase chain reaction (PCR) which was used to identify the species of meat present in a sample. The initial tests revealed unknown DNA to be present. A second round of PCR testing was conducted which was specific for three meat species (bovine, porcine, and equine). The results highlighted that one-third of the samples contained equine DNA and 80% contained porcine DNA, but were declared on pack as beef.

The FSAI made their report public in January 2013 and the media and industry in the United Kingdom and Europe quickly picked up the story. Foods standards authorities, consumer groups, and the media started to sample and test the authenticity of beef containing foods both branded and own label.

The industry was also galvanized into testing their products and the integrity of their beef and other meat supply chains. Initial tests revealed that frozen entree's (lasagne, spaghetti bolognaise) supplied by a large European comaker for major supermarket chains' own branded products and branded products contained significant quantities of horse meat - in one instance, a 100% horse meat instead of beef.

The immediate impact

Trust in the food industry as a whole was immediately compromised and a major study by Which in March 2013 showed that 6 out of every 10 consumers had changed their shopping habits with regard to processed foods. Consumer groups, retailers, and food service outlets sought assurance from their suppliers to guarantee the authenticity of meat-containing products. This was initially confined to fresh and frozen products but quickly spread to ambient stable products.

Analytical capacity for PCR testing quickly became scarce with lead times moved from 3 to 4 days to several weeks at a price premium.

What follows is a brief account of the experience of one major branded food manufacturer during this time of crisis for the industry as a whole and the steps taken to identify the risks within their supply chain and the controls required in the future to ensure supply chain integrity and ingredient authenticity.

Meat supply chain integrity and risk

At the start of the crisis, a global task force was established and led by the chief quality officer, comprising procurement, country and regional supply chain, external affairs, legal, and country and regional quality management. Both the initial report from the FSAI and follow-up assessments from the UK FSA indicated that fresh and frozen beef had been targeted in a major trading standards fraud.

Given the findings indicated that the fraud was confined to fresh and frozen beef products, the initial crisis team's technical view was that it was unlikely that our products had been affected by the fraud, given the vast majority of our business was in ambient stable products. However, we required robust evidence that this was actually the case, given adulteration of highly processed meat and meat derivatives such as meat powders, pastes, and stock would be relatively easy and very hard to identify without the use of PCR testing techniques.

A review of fresh, frozen, dehydrated, and processed meat supply chains was initiated going back to the slaughterhouse and in some cases back to the farm.

While the focus of the media and the authorities was fresh and frozen comminuted beef products, it was clear to the task force that meat and meat derivatives were widely used in dehydrated soups, entrees, and bouillons and that many of the upstream processes from first-tier (suppliers of raw materials to the business) and second-tier (suppliers to the first-tier suppliers) suppliers all had the potential to incorporate mixed species. While all suppliers were required to be certified by Global Food Safety Initiative (GFSI) recognized standards, in 2013, there was no mandatory requirement within those standards to implement food security risk assessments such as Carver and Shock and apply controls for high-risk items.

The task force identified high-, medium-, and low supply chain risks based on the origin of the meat processed by Tier 1 and Tier 2 suppliers.

- High risk - meat and meat derivatives composed of materials that have been bought on the spot market or from traders and other vendors.
- Medium risk - meat and meat derivatives composed of materials that have been purchased direct from a slaughterhouse which operated across a range of meat species.
- Low risk - meat and meat derivatives arising from an integrated supply chain.

That is a dedicated slaughterhouse dealing in single species or dealing in multispecies but the individual operations are fully segregated.

A secondary set of risk criteria was also used within the risk assessment. This included an assessment by our meat technical and commercial experts as to whether the materials were sufficiently visually distinct to be a robust means of identification in our inbound supply. For example, any comminuted meat product is by definition not visually distinct and therefore generally considered to be high risk. However, this risk rating could be moderated if the supply chain was fully integrated back to the slaughterhouse and the slaughterhouse was either dedicated to a single species or had fully segregated meat processing unit operations.

A series of detailed supplier requirements were defined which can be summarized as follows:

- First-tier and second-tier suppliers that are single species do not need PCR test.
- First-tier and second-tier suppliers that handle and provide visually distinct materials do not need PCR test.
- All suppliers must have validated and monitored cleaning procedures between meat species.
- First-tier and second-tier suppliers that are multispecies and/or supply non- visually distinct materials must take the PCR test and provide a certificate of analysis (CoA) with all dispatches.
- First-tier suppliers that are multispecies and produce dehydrated powders and pastes/stocks that have heat processes which do not fully degrade DNA must take the PCR test and provide a CoA with all dispatches. If the DNA is proven to be fully degraded, no PCR testing is required.

This latter point must first be agreed and approved by quality management.

- All company manufacturing sites will carry out PCR testing on the first six lots from all meat suppliers who supply nonvisually distinct materials where the DNA has not been degraded. If all six lots pass successfully, then random skip lot sampling can commence. Any failure must be resolved and requalification through first six-lot PCR testing should be initiated.

The first six lots were chosen because it is the lowest statistically significant number of sequential events that can occur without it being down to random pure chance.

The company crisis team also stipulated that seven species PCR (beef, horse, chicken, turkey, pig, goat, and sheep) test must be carried by suppliers at an external laboratory that was accredited and certified to ISO 17025 for that method.

Details of these now standard requirements were communicated to each supplier and a database was established to include supplier, supplier location, raw material and number, raw material location, risk assessment level, tiered level, whether a certificate of conformance (CoC) or a certificate of analysis (CoA) was required, and whether to be supplied in advance or with shipments. Where a CoA was required, these materials had to be positively released on the basis of the data on the CoA.

As stated earlier, all meat powders, pastes, stocks, meat derivative compound ingredients including flavors were considered nonvisually distinct in terms of meat species content and thus required the first six lots in bound to be tested using PCR seven species at accredited laboratories. All suppliers of raw materials were required to use the same approach on their raw meat supplies based on the risk assessments from their respective upstream supply chains.

It's worth noting that meat stocks and pastes are highly processed with heat and pressure and it was quickly established that any DNA present was too degraded to give any viable results from PCR testing. Where this was the case, suppliers were required to be able to demonstrate that the materials used in stock preparation were not contaminated or adulterated with other meat species, via the use of chain of custody evidence along their respective supply chains.

The global task force defined how our own manufacturing operations and those of our copackers must handle meat and meat derivative supplies. All operations were made aware of the risk assessment and tier level of the supplier and raw material and the requirement for appropriate action to be implemented such as the following:

- Visual identification accompanied with a CoC.
- The requirement for a CoA of seven species PCR testing from a certified external laboratory from supplier and first six-lot sampling and testing by the sourcing units (with the raw material lot on positive release), moving to skip lot once the first six lots were confirmed as free from contamination.

Sourcing unit inbound samples were sent off to the approved laboratories. The results were collated centrally using the database and lots communicated for release or appropriate action to the sourcing units.

Details of the supplier CoC were also entered into the database by the sourcing unit.

For third party manufacturing (copackers/comakers), a similar approach was mandated in terms of risk assessment, tier levels, and implementation of six-lot positive release for each appropriate raw material. Again, their results were collated centrally and reported through the centralized database.

Customer and authority communication and testing

The global task force agreed that the testing of finished products should not be carried out. The rationale being that testing of finished products did not offer any benefit in the identification and elimination of adulterated raw materials from the supply chain.

This rationale was communicated to all customers and the authorities with mixed responses from those customers who expected a CoA for finished goods, particularly in the food service sector. Lobbying top to top was frequently required to allow supply of finished goods to customers based on the analytical results from raw material testing. All deliveries were accompanied by a CoC. PCR results could be supplied on request, but this was rarely needed.

With the positive assurance approach and the databases of results, it was possible to verify and communicate compliance throughout our supply chain.

Analytical methods

During the meat adulteration scandal, the two most common commercially accessible techniques for meat speciation testing were ELISA (enzyme-linked immuno- sorbent assay) and PCR, detecting species-specific animal proteins or DNA targets, respectively.

With the need to evaluate a range of raw and processed meat/meat-derived materials, PCR offered most in respect of sensitivity, the ability to detect a broader range of different meat species, and applicability to both raw and processed materials. ELISA methods at the time were mostly limited to detection of raw meat species, with process induced damage to the target proteins rendering processed meat materials undetected/unquantifiable by ELISA.

The PCR method used to evaluate raw materials identified for testing by risk assessment enabled sensitive screening for the presence of seven meat species (beef, horse, chicken, turkey, pig, goat, and sheep) at or above 0.1% w/w and where contamination was detected to quantify (limit of quantitation 0.5%-1.0% w/w) whether the contamination was at a level suggesting cross contamination (<1.0%), poor management of integrity at the supplier (1%-5%)), or potential adulteration. 1% was defined by the authorities as a pragmatic short-term benchmark for acceptable cross contamination.

During the evaluation of meat/meat-derived raw materials, it quickly became clear that great care is needed in understanding both the applicability of methods to specific materials and in interpretation of results, for example:

- Extensive processing of meat materials (e.g., high-temperature, long-heat process) degrades the DNA, rendering the presence of a meat material as non-detectable or significantly underreported by PCR testing. If meat components present in a raw material have been processed differently, their relative proportions identified in testing may be skewed, with the contaminant species either underreported or overestimated, depending on which of the host or contaminant species has been most impacted by processing.

- Different meat species and different meat tissues contain differing amounts of DNA, especially of mitochondrial DNA, potentially impacting respective quantitation in a mixture. Nuclear DNA is more consistent in level between species and tissues and can offer a better target for quantitative analysis.
- The analytical recovery of DNA from different species/ tissues may not be the same in extraction prior to PCR testing.

It is important therefore to understand as much as possible about the test materials and potential meat "contaminants" present and to work with the test laboratory to understand potential issues in testing/quantitation, whether testing is likely to be meaningful and what options exist to mitigate issues in testing, such as the use of appropriate control samples.

Discussion and key learnings

- Ensure that any incident crisis team includes key functions such as legal and external affairs in addition to other technical functions.
- All external communications must be approved by the central crisis team and other senior stakeholders before release. Any local requests for local needs must be clearly communicated to and agreed by the central team.
- Ensure that all internal senior stakeholders are updated frequently with results, current status, and future actions. There should be no surprises and everyone should be fully aligned on the process and the progress.
- Work constructively with high-risk suppliers (including copackers) and their supply chains to establish pragmatic controls which can be easily managed without excessive costs.

- Ensure that suppliers which use frozen raw materials that could vary widely in age (in some instances up to 2 years) are included within the risk assessment and any testing regime.
- Recognize the risks of buying materials on the spot market where origins and provenance are unclear and where necessary eliminate that as a source of supply.
- Review the adulteration risk of all high value raw materials and put plans in place to verify authenticity. Ensure that the risk assessment tools going forward include geopolitical factors which can sometimes drive adulteration risks.
- Ensure that all stakeholders understand the regulations with regard to materials contamination and use of that material in a formulation and the subsequent dilution of the contaminant. "Dilution is not the solution to the pollution" in the eyes of the law and the authorities.
- Establish and understand in detail the key differences between the limit of detection and the limit of quantitation for the methods being used and the implications of results between the two this has from a regulatory perspective vis-à-vis release decision due diligence.
- Test methods have continued to improve since the horse meat scandal.

Commercially available PCR testing offers both increased sensitivity, being able to screen for meat species at 0.01% contamination, and an extended range of target meat species. However, current and future developments in DNA sequencing methods, such as NGS (next-generation sequencing), offer a step forward in testing capability. NGS uses parallel sequencing to enable many thousands of DNA fragments to be sequenced simultaneously, in principle allowing identification of all DNA containing meat (and other) species present in a meat (food) sample. The technology relies on access to comprehensive reference gene databases and availability of reliable species-specific primers. Of course, NGS technology also relies on the presence of intact nondegraded DNA in the meat components present and faces the same challenges as outlined earlier for PCR testing; the relative proportions of species DNA identified may not align with the quantitative proportions of different meat materials present. Improved options are also available for ELISA-based speciation testing.

Methods based on detection of heat-resistant glycoproteins have improved detectability of cooked/processed meat materials, although detection of extensively processed materials remains difficult. The species scope of commercially available ELISA test options remains much more limited by comparison to DNA technologies. Rapid lateral flow devices for detection of raw meat species (pork, beef, sheep, poultry, horse) are now available for routine QC at suppliers processing raw meat, allowing immediate assurance at intake and/or validation of internal integrity controls.

Note

- First-tier supplier is a supplier to the company.
- Second-tier supplier is a supplier to the first-tier suppliers.
- Third-tier supplier is a supplier to the second-tier suppliers.

8.4 Counterfeit mayonnaise

Some employees of a food manufacturing site in a South American country walked across a local market when they saw a small vendor stall with jars of mayonnaise, labeled as their company's product and in the correct size jars, but priced well below normal levels. They bought a few jars. The product inside indeed appeared to be mayonnaise, but did not quite have the correct color or consistency.

Further investigation revealed that this was not the company's own product, although the labels, jars, and lids all appeared to be authentic. Microbiological tests of the product did not indicate any discernible microbial risk, but chemical risks could not be excluded, since the origin of the oil and other ingredients was not known. All in all, this looked like a simple case of counterfeit product and action had to be taken in order to protect the brand and not give – implicit - license to counterfeiters. The police were informed with a request to remove the product from the market, but not to prosecute the vendors, who were presumed to be local and economically challenged. Authorities took action as requested and things went quiet for a couple of months.

Then the story repeated itself - jars with mayonnaise and somewhat outdated but nevertheless authentic labels were offered on the same marketplace. It was clear that simply removing the product from the market was not enough to stop the operation, but local police were not interested in further investigations, so the company involved their own security professionals.

They found the place where the counterfeit product was made - a garage in town. It took some more investigating but then they also found where the labels had come from. This was an inside job. Old label material that was no longer used and was destined to be destroyed was actually sold by a factory employee to the counterfeiters. Lastly, there was the question where the jars and caps came from. Finally, it was discovered that the counterfeiters salvaged jars and caps from the local landfill, which were then washed by hand. Since this provided only limited numbers of jars/caps, "production" of counterfeit mayonnaise was also limited.

No single definitive source for the oil and other ingredients was determined -the operation appeared to be scavenging around for anything that was available at the time.

Discussion and key learnings

- Destruction of rejected or outdated materials needs to be witnessed and certified.
- Counterfeit operations always need to be fully investigated, especially if original materials appear to be part of the counterfeit product.
- Although no food safety risk was immediately identified, the full picture of the production process of the counterfeit product would suggest that this product could never be regarded as safe.
- A regular informal inspection of local markets in countries where cottage industry counterfeiting is not uncommon makes sense.

Chapter Nine

Dangerous products - or are they?

9.1 The memory of a mushroom poisoning

In my professional lifetime, I have experienced different types of intoxications. Here is a case of mushroom intoxication which affected an entire family.

In June 2014, seven people from the same family, including a 2-year-old child, got intoxicated after eating a green-spored parasol mushroom (Chlorophyllum molybdites), a wild grown mushroom, picked in the garden behind the house. Within an hour after eating the mushroom, they suffered symptoms of abdominal pain, nausea, vomiting, and diarrhoea.

The patients were promptly given first aid. They were asked to drink activated charcoal, infusion, gastric lavage, and then transferred to a nearby Poison Prevention Center Hospital for follow-up treatment. After 1 week, all patients including the 2-year-old child were in stable condition, and the story ended happily.

Immediately after receiving the news of the poisoning case, the Food Hygiene and Safety Department of the Ministry of Health in collaboration with health authorities in the area updated their public health information and communication link. This in order to raise awareness of poisonous mushrooms in the community.

Discussion and key learnings

In some countries, mushrooms are an essential element in the daily diet and therefore people regularly pick mushrooms for consumption in wild natural areas. Naturally, they try to avoid poisonous mushrooms as these can be very dangerous, but recognizing them can be difficult and there are many misperceptions around:

- Some people think that poisonous mushrooms are typically colorful, but in the northern provinces of our country, there are deadly poisonous mushrooms that are of a pure white color.
- Some people think that mushrooms that are eaten by insects are not poisonous, but some toxins that humans are vulnerable to have no effect on insects, worms, ants, or snails.
- Regrettably, some people try to feed their domestic animals first and if the animals don't die, they conclude that the mushrooms are not poisonous, but this is only true for some mushrooms and some animals, as many animal species, are not sensitive to gastrointestinal toxins. Moreover, in some cases, it takes 12 h after eating mushrooms to show the first symptoms and affected animals usually die at 5-7 days after eating poisonous mushrooms.
- Some people even "test" their mushrooms with silver spoons or chopsticks, in the expectation that they will see a color change if the mushroom is poisonous, but that is a wholly unreliable method.

Therefore, where picking and consumption of wild mushrooms is common, the public should be educated to recognize poisonous mushrooms, every mushroom season again. They should also learn to recognize signs of mushroom poisoning and the need to immediately consult health professionals.

Further reading

The following references are originally in Vietnamese. Online translation available.

- https://www.chongdoc.org.vn/ngo-doc-nam-43452.
- http://soytetuyenquang.gov.vn/tin-tuc-su-kien/an-toan-thuc-

pham/ngo-doc-thuc-pham/ngo-doc-nam-doc-cach-xu-tri-va-dieu-tri.html.

- https://www.vinmec.com/vi/tin-tuc/thong-tin-suc-khoe/suc-khoe-tong-quat/dieu-tri-ngo-doc- nam-doc/.

9.2 Say "no" to puffer fish

In my professional life, I have witnessed many cases of poisoning due to consumption of puffer fish. Repeatedly, consumers are warned not to eat these fish because of the highly dangerous toxins in the meat. Still, people continue to ignore the recommendations and puffer fish poisoning remains a recurring event, leading to fatalities.

In October 2017, six fishermen were hospitalized because of food poisoning caused by eating puffer fish they caught. They showed signs of food poisoning such as convulsions, vomiting, defecation, and respiratory failure.

The patients were taken to an emergency room, but one died of severe poisoning before reaching the hospital. The other five were given first aid and remained in critical condition for a while. In this case, thanks to timely treatment, all their lives were saved.

In another case, in March 2018, there were five patients poisoned by eating puffer fish they had caught and cooked. An hour later, the patients experienced stiff limbs, stiff jaws, could not speak, and had to be hospitalized in a state of deep coma, cardiac arrest, apnoea, low blood pressure. The patients were actively resuscitated, intubated, and respirated. Two patients regained consciousness later while the remaining three patients were comatose and continued to require mechanical respiration. After intensive treatment all patients recovered.

Discussion and key learnings

Puffer fish meat contains a neurotoxin (tetrodotoxin) that has great heat stability and a high mortality rate (up to 60% if emergency treatment is slow). Causes of death are paralysis of the respiratory muscles and hypotension. The puffer fish toxin is 1200 times more potent than cyanide; less than 2 mg of the toxin can kill a person and one mature puffer fish is enough to kill 30 people.

Boiling at a temperature of 100∘C for 6 h only reduces tetrodotoxin by 50%, and the toxin only completely disappears when boiling at 200∘C for 10 min. Therefore, it is impossible to lose the toxicity of puffer fish by normal cooking and processing.

Up to now, there is no specific treatment for tetrodotoxin poisoning. Therefore, to prevent puffer fish poisoning, the most effective measure is not to eat any food that is made from or has been in contact with puffer fish: "say no to puffer fish".

Further reading

The following references are originally in Vietnamese. Online translation available.

- https://vinmec.com/vi/tin-tuc/thong-tin-suc-khoe/suc-khoe-tong-quat/ngo-doc-ca-noc-nguyen-nhan-dau-hieu.
- http://antoanthucpham.quangtri.gov.vn/Tin-tuc-su-kien/ngo-doc-thuc-pham-do-ca-noc-va- cach-phong-tranh-1173.html.
- http://bachmai.gov.vn/tin-tuc-va-su-kien/y-hoc-thuong-thuc-menuleft-32/4244-hiem-hoa-khon-luong-khi-che-bien-mon-an-tu-ca-noc.html.

9.3 Oil safety story in Taiwan

In 1979, a lot of small abscesses suddenly started appearing on the faces of all students of a school for disabled children. At first, the teacher suspected that the problem was caused by the meals. However, extensive investigations revealed no clues. This teacher did not give up and continued the investigations. Finally, through a cooperation with a hospital, the issue was traced to rice oil.

During the deodorization step of the refining process of rice oil, the heating elements were leaking and the heating medium-polychlorinated biphenyl (PCB) was leaking into the rice oil.
An outbreak of PCB poisoning from the consumption of contaminated rice oil, covering four counties in central Taiwan, was investigated. There were 1843 cases by the end of 1980. The highest frequency of incidence occurred during the period from March to July 1979. The severity of clinical manifestations varied. Most patients showed symptoms of mild or moderate severity. The major age group affected was between 11 and 20 years old. Most of the victims were students and factory workers. The amount of PCB intake in each victim was estimated to be 0.7-1.84 g and the latent period from the time of intake to the onset of clinical manifestations was approximately 3-4 months.

The PCB accident caused the death of 16 people and injured 2000. Early in 1968, the same had also happened in Japan and PCB was no longer used there. All victims and their offspring next generation are still on medication until this day, in accordance with a specific law (health care law of oil victims). I am the medical doctor prescribing the medication for them and their next generation. The image is deeply and greatly impressed in my mind.

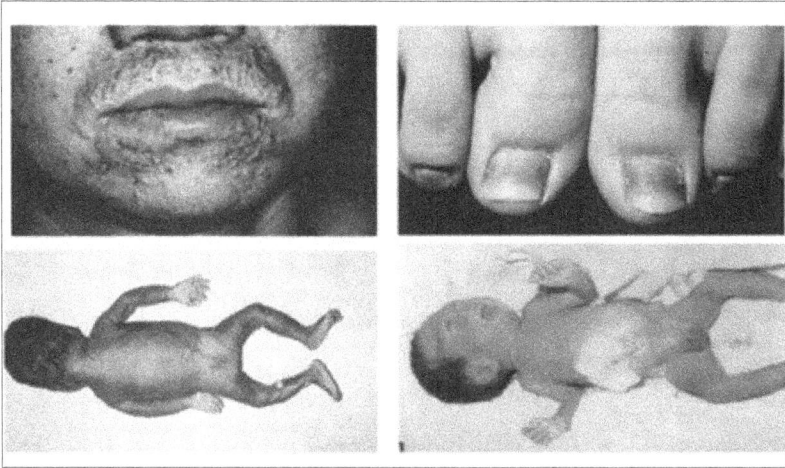

Fig. 9.3.1 The syndrome for PCB rice oil victim

In 2013 (34 years after the PCB oil event), adulterated olive oil was found in the market. High amounts of commercial chlorophylls in an oil factory caused this event. The added amounts of chlorophyll (food additives) were very low, but the idea of fraud involving - very high priced - olive oil was still very scary for consumers. The worst was in 2014. Recycled cooking oil and gutter oil were refined again and sold in the market (Fig. 9.3.2). A farmer noticed a very bad smell around his farm, and after a long process of tracing and evidence collection, the serious and terrible oil problem was found. The company involved was prosecuted and heavily fined.

In 2017, national law adopted an anonymous whistleblower's clause. Government encourages the employees of food and beverage industries to report the potential food safety problem or any illegal process or the addition of unauthorized materials. In addition, all whistleblowers are completely protected. After evaluation, a whistleblower could get a reward (20% of the total value of the sold products) if the allegations are found to be true. As a result, there were several cases where employees stepped forward and "blew the whistle" on the misuse of expired oil and some other fraud events. This has had a very positive impact on food safety, which is now much better supported.

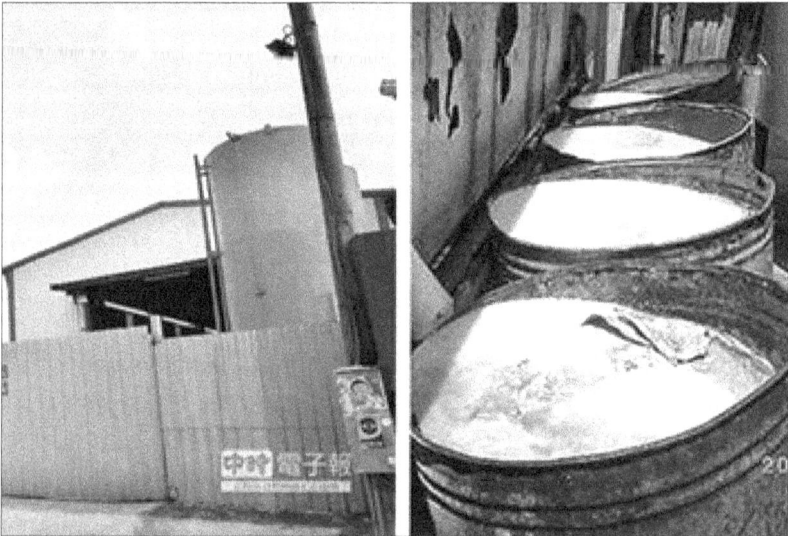

Fig 9.3.2 Gutter oil factory

Discussion and key learnings

- Food safety incidents will continue to happen. We will never completely eliminate them.
- Some food safety incidents could have been prevented, if the government had put effective monitoring systems in place.
- The introduction of effective whistleblower encouragement and protection legislation has helped in detecting and containing food safety incidents.
- There should never be only a very thin wall between a food product and a harmful substance - as in heat exchangers.

Further reading

- Five-point Food Safety Policy, 2019. Department of Information Services. Executive Yuan, Taiwan.
- Hsu, S.T., Ma, C.I., Hsu, S.K., Wu, S.S., Hsu, N.H., Yeh, C.C., Wu, S.B., 1985. Discovery and epidemiology of PCB poisoning in Taiwan: a four-year follow-up. Environ. Health Perspect. 59, 5-10.
- Motarjemi, Y., June 2014. Whistleblowing: Food Safety and Fraud. Food Safety Magazine. https://www.food-safety.com/articles/3670-whistleblowing-food-safety-and-fraud.
- Motarjemi, Y., 2023. Whistleblowing: an essential element of public health and food safety management. In: Andersen, V., Lelieveld, H., Motarjemi, Y. (Eds.), Food Safety Management. A Practical Guide for the Food Industry, second ed. Academic Press. Waltham MA.
- Reggiani, G., Bruppacher, R., 1985. Symptoms, signs and findings in humans exposed to PCBs and their derivatives. Environ. Health Perspect. 60, 225-232.

9.4 Bufotoxin poisoning caused by eating toad meat

One day in April 2020, I learned that four six- to eight-year-old kids had been hospitalized because of toad poisoning. It was reported by the children's family that while playing with other kids, the children caught and then grilled toads for their meals. An hour after eating the toads, the children were found to vomit and were taken to an emergency room for treatment. The most serious patient exhibited a range of symptoms: vomiting, lethargy, slow heart rate, difficulty with breathing. In another case, in October 2020, three sisters were hospitalized for treatment because of toad poisoning. After noticing symptoms of nausea, abdominal pain and diarrhoea, the family took these three to a hospital. The sisters had caught some toads and eggs, cooked and ate them. They found the toad eggs good; however, they all developed symptoms of dizziness, nausea and diarrhoea shortly afterward. Before going to the hospital, they made an effort to vomit to lose as much the poison they could. This action helped them a speedy recovery.

Discussion and key learnings

Despite frequent warnings regarding toad poisoning, many people in my country still catch and cook toads for their meals, and end up being poisoned. Toad meat does contain several nutrients, and is being used in traditional medicine, especially for rickets in children, but toads need to be prepared and processed carefully and skillfully because they may lead to serious illness and fatalities.

The toxic ingredient in toad is bufotoxin, an extremely toxic substance, found in the liver, eggs and skin as a milky white secretion from the glands under the skin, parotid, in the eyes and in the nerve ganglia of the toad, causing symptoms such as nausea, vomiting, pain and bloating, diarrhoea, heart rhythm disturbances, drop in blood pressure, shock, hallucinations, and headache. In serious cases, patient's liver and kidney can be damaged. If not treated immediately, it can kill people in a very short time. It is estimated that the amount of bufotoxin in one mature toad can kill four to five healthy people, and children are especially at risk.

Further reading

The following references are originally in Vietnamese. Online translation available.

- https://soyte.namdinh.gov.vn/home/hoat-dong-nganh/giao-duc-suc-khoe/cach-phong-tranh-ngo-doc-khi-su-dung-thit-coc. https://bvndtp.org.vn/nhung-cau-hoi-ve-thit-coc-loi-va-hai/
- http://bachmai.gov.vn/tin-noi-bat/41-tin-noi-bat/1068-ngo-doc-vi-an-thit-coc-1068.html

9.5 Goat liver with "Arak": a controversial myth

During spring break, I decided to invite a colleague who had joined us from abroad over for a traditional Lebanese lunch. One of the delicacies in this diet is raw goat liver, cut into small pieces, which is consumed along with the traditional alcoholic beverage, the "Arak". Like any other raw food, there are special recommendations to be followed in order for the meal to be healthy and safe. It is known that this food might carry a parasite, Dicrocoelium lanceatum, which lives in the bile ducts of infected cattle, and may thus reach their liver. A good butcher can determine whether a liver is safe or not; and a local myth says that drinking alcohol while eating raw goat liver will kill any potential parasite.

The food was served in a very presentable manner. During mid-meal, I felt a tingling feeling in my throat, a swelling and feeling of choking with a difficult cough. At that moment, I knew that I had consumed a potentially infected liver piece. I was advised to drink more "Arak" to kill the parasite or dislodge it from my throat. I did not do that and as my situation got worse, I clearly needed medical intervention. I was rushed to the hospital where I was given cortisone injection to relieve the pain and reduce the inflammation along with a specific medication, which helps to eliminate the parasite in the digestive tract. After I started feeling better, the health provider jokingly said that it was a wise decision to seek medical attention rather than sipping more "Arak," as recommended by the myth, since it would only cause a hangover and not solve the problem.

Thankfully, the infected piece of goat liver was my share; otherwise, it would have been very unpleasant hospitality service for our international guest.

Discussion and key learnings

In this case, five main food safety principles apply:

- People need to understand that raw meat is an inherently risky product,
- Raw goat liver needs to be inspected by food specialists and kept at proper refrigeration, and
- Inspections need to cover the entire chain from farm to fork. The animals also need to be checked for any possible infections before proceeding to the consumption phase.
- The butcher/food handler should have been more aware of the risk associated with consuming such food and consequently abide by the official guidelines, and
- Consumers should rely on scientific evidence rather than on myths like drinking alcohol to avoid infection.

Further reading

- Dicrocoeliasis, 2019. Content Source: Global Health, Division of Parasitic Diseases and Malaria. CDC.
- Ta¸s Cengiz, Z., Yilmaz, H., Cumhur Du¨lger, A., C¸ ic¸ekc, M., March-April 2010. Human infection with Dicrocoelium dendriticum in Turkey. Ann. Saudi. Med. 30 (2), 159-161. https://doi.org/10.4103/0256-4947.60525.

9.6 Risk with glass jars

The packaged food industry is constantly looking for new product ideas that will grow their business. Sometimes, what looks like a blockbuster new item turns out to be a disaster. Take the case of the ornate "snowman jar" filled with a thick confectionery product. The jar is glass shaped like a snowman. Covering the glass jar is a colorful printed plastic jacket displaying a snowman complete with coal buttons and eyes of coal, etc. The plastic cap on the jar is in the shape of a top hat. The jar is designed to be washed out and used as a decoration or for storage of candies or nuts, etc. Great idea! Top management loves it.

Unfortunately, shortly after introduction to the marketplace, complaints, through the company's consumer contact line, started coming in that consumers were finding broken glass when they scooped out the product. There were also some cases of injury! It was clear that there was a serious design problem in glass manufacturing or through the filling and distribution processes. A large recall of all distributed product was undertaken.

Jars returned for analysis revealed impact breaks under the decorative plastic jacket covering the jar. This could have occurred any time from manufacturing of the glass jars themselves through filling and distribution to the consumer. The problem is that if an impact break occurs, the thick product will not visibly leak. The plastic wrap holds it in. At the consumer, the product is scooped from the jar and the broken glass, imbedded in the thick product, is scooped up with it.

Discussion and key learnings

Research and Development product developers and packaging suppliers need a process to assess physical risks from product packaging design. No risk assessment was done in this case. Had the product been a free-flowing liquid, the issue would have been evident sooner. In this case, it was not.

This company learned about the problem shortly after the introduction of the product. Receiving and being able to react promptly to complaints is essential in being able to manage a developing incident situation. This requires a robust consumer contact system that is easy to use (i.e., a toll-free number) so that issues can be brought to the quality/food safety staff quickly. In addition, an alert protocol for serious complaint escalation (i.e., illness, injury, etc.) needs to be in place to alert them immediately versus a minor complaint such as off flavor or color.

Learnings from incidents such as this must be shared with the food and glass manufacturing industries to prevent reoccurrence.

9.7 Salmonellosis outbreak during a religious feast

In Catholic countries and regions, the Feast of Corpus Christi is celebrated 60 days after Easter, typically in June. In our rural area, too, this day has a long tradition and is the most important religious holiday of the year. The population wears historic dresses and stays together all day after the mass and procession with food, drink, and games.

In one community, the women of the village made their own mayonnaise for the communal lunch. At end of the day, the leftover mayonnaise was distributed to different families, as there is nothing better than homemade products.

A few days later, all members of a family fell ill with salmonellosis. No other illnesses occurred within this community.

In subsequent investigations and analyses, the pathogen was detected in all leftover mayonnaise; however, in the sample taken from the affected family, it was found at high concentration.

It is thought that the salmonella contamination was probably coming from raw eggs or an infected but symptomless person, preparing the mayonnaise. Of course, cross-contamination cannot be excluded either. The exact route of contamination could never be identified. However, it was found that the affected family had not refrigerated the mayonnaise. That year, June was particularly hot and provided optimal conditions for the growth of Salmonella.

Discussion and key learnings

The obvious cardinal error is that the mayonnaise was not kept refrigerated, for several days. Combined with inadequate acidity, Salmonella was able to multiply to concentrations above the minimum infective dose. Refrigeration is among one of the most important operations to ensure food safety. This example shows how a single mistake can lead to foodborne illness.

The story also underpins the limitations of regulatory controls in preventing foodborne diseases, as they cannot operate in the household setting or informal sector. To effectively prevent foodborne disease, food control must be combined with consumer health education. This education could start early in life, for example, in schools.

Further reading

- ICMSF, 1996. Microorganisms in Foods 5: Characteristics of Pathogens.
- Motarjemi, Y., 2014. Public health measures: health education, information, and risk communication. In: Encyclopedia of Food Safety, vol. 4. Elsevier, pp. 123-132.

9.8 Warm chicken, or why management attitude determines safe food

In some Asian countries the general expectation is for meat to be eaten fresh or warm. This applies in particular for chicken where consumers expect a bird freshly slaughtered is the best quality. Hence, the birds are purchased and slaughtered in a local market and taken home or to the restaurant for immediate cooking. Sales of commercial chilled chicken are relatively small as the consumer trust is not established.

The retailer I worked for wanted to sell warm chicken in the chilled department, and to demonstrate how fresh the carcasses were, they would be sold with smears of blood and feces on them. Just like how they appear freshly slaughtered in the market albeit they are obviously cleaned immediately afterward before cooking.

As a respected international brand, selling meat like this was a no-go. But the new managing director of the local business insisted it went ahead, and a long and drawn- out process of convincing him this was not the right thing began. The matter was escalated, making him dig in his heels. He simply refused to understand why this was an issue despite the best efforts of the Quality Assurance (QA) department to convince him. So, the QA and customer management departments worked together to inform and educate the customers as to the freshness of the chickens sold. The customers were shown how the chickens were processed by a specially developed local supplier nearby, chilled at the supplier to keep them fresh and delivered within a tight timeframe to the store. Restaurant and catering clients could have them delivered directly. The quality would be the right level for their needs and they would be safe.

After many months of customer engagement, the chicken sales went ahead and there were no carcasses with feces nor blood in the chilled section. The managing director was not with the company for long afterward.

Discussion and key learnings

- Assumed common sense hygiene practices don't necessarily translate to different operating environments. Understanding the local customs and finding a way to operate while maintaining safety is essential to gain long term goodwill.
- Customer engagement is a long process and it takes time to build trust. Face to face discussions are needed when a completely new concept is introduced.
- Quality and food safety functions can do an excellent job of securing a brand's reputation when they work well with commercial departments to engage and educate customers.

Further reading

- Motarjemi, Y., Ross, T. Risk analysis: risk communication: biological hazards, In: Encyclopedia of Food Safety, Elsevier.
- WHO, 2000. Foodborne Disease, a Focus on Health Education. World Health Organziation, Geneva.

9.9 A mysterious outbreak of "sleeping sickness" in Angola

An outbreak of acute neurological disease of unknown origin occurred from October to December 2007 in Cacuaco Municipality, Angola, which has a population of about 1.3 million. The most distinguishing symptom was that victims were falling asleep and could only be aroused through painful stimulation. Other symptoms included extreme somnolence, persistent drowsiness, blurred vision, difficulty speaking, and loss of muscle control. It was reported that some dogs and chickens were also falling asleep. Patients recovered slowly over a number of days but many still had difficulty walking. The disease would ultimately affect 467 individuals - a majority of whom were children. The original "sleeping sickness" is caused by a parasite transmitted by the tsetse fly, but this disease was clearly not East African trypanosomiasis as other symptoms did not match and the vector was not present.

The first cases occurred in early October and were officially reported on 24 October to the Angolan Ministry of Health (AMOH). Shortly thereafter, the World Health Organization (WHO) country office, in cooperation with the AMOH, conducted initial investigations. Although the cause could not be identified, the symptoms suggested that this was an intoxication rather than an infection. On October 30, 2007, the AMOH officially requested WHO to provide experts to investigate this outbreak. Most of the information in this chapter is taken from the Executive Summary of the report prepared by this team of experts (Gutschmidt et al., 2008).

The WHO team arrived in the country on 2 November, consisting of a clinical toxicologist, an epidemiologist, an environmental investigator, a laboratory specialist, and a team coordinator. In collaboration with the national authorities, some members of the team set about identifying the cause of the outbreak through the clinical and neurological examinations of more than 50 patients. This included taking blood and urine samples that were shipped to laboratories in Europe. The neurological examination reported:

"Patients had extreme somnolence. On awakening they had ataxia,1 lasting several days. The central nervous system (CNS) was affected, particularly the cerebellum (altered balance and coordination). All other vital parameters were normal. In particular, there was no sign of peripheral neuropathy. No vomiting nor diarrhoea were consistently reported. Differential diagnosis supported a toxic origin, likely through a substance affecting the gamma-aminobutyric acid (GABA)-receptors." Consequently, benzodiazepines in the water supply were initial suspected.

Other team members conducted an epidemiological investigation to identify the source of the outbreak, including the collection of food and water samples, which were also sent to laboratories in Europe for analysis. Children under 15 years of age were the largest group affected (64%) followed by females (62%). Some evidence indicated household clusters but not all members were affected. Bacterial or viral infections were not indicated by the epidemiological curve and interviews did not point to a common source of exposure. Samples of blood and urine were taken and sent to laboratories in Germany and the United Kingdom. The samples were tested for more than 7000 substances, including benzodiazepines, gammahydroxybutyrate analogs, pharmaceutical and metabolites, organic solvents, and heavy metals.

On 19 November, the laboratory in Germany detected very high concentrations of bromide ranging from 1000-2450 mg/L in six out of seven blood samples, 20-50 times higher than normal physiological levels. On 21 November, the laboratory in the United Kingdom confirmed these findings in a different set of blood samples, which showed similarly high bromide levels. It should be noted that although three deaths were reported earlier, the cause of these deaths was later determined to be unrelated to bromide. Food and water samples collected on the field were then tested for bromide in Germany and Switzerland. In particular, analysis of four out of six table salt samples was shown to contain at least 80% of sodium bromide. Two other food items that were in contact with this salt were also found positive for bromide. Altogether, these laboratory results strongly indicated that ingestion of "table salt" (that actually was mostly sodium bromide) produced the neurological symptoms observed among cases.

As a result of these findings, risk management activities were initiated, including informing the public about the potential risk of "table salt" and providing healthcare facilities advice on treatment. In addition, testing of salt was initiated using a simple analytical method. The WHO team made recommendations to prevent and respond to further incidents, including the strengthening of national chemical and food safety programs and establishing a national poison center with associated clinical and analytical toxicological capacities. Although sodium bromide is used in Angola in the oil industry to make a heavy clear brine for drilling, it is still unknown how sodium bromide came to be substituted for table salt.

Discussion and key learnings

The lesson from this unusual outbreak is that the investigation of possible chemical etiology should be conducted in a systematic manner. In this regard, WHO advice has been recently updated (WHO, 2021). In any investigation of unknown etiology, food should be considered a potential vehicle until it can be explicitly ruled out.

Ideally, such investigations should include an epidemiologist familiar with foodborne investigation and control (WHO, 2008).

Given the large number of potential hazards in food and the urgency of ongoing outbreaks, investigations could be expedited by an international database of individual outbreaks, including summarized (1) location of the event, (2) clinical data, (3) epidemiologic data, (4) laboratory findings, and (5) results of on-site investigations (Guzewich et al., 1997).

References

- Gutschmidt, K., Haefliger, P., Zilker, T., 2008. Outbreak of neurological illness of unknown etiology in Cacuaco Municipality, Angola, Executive Summary, WHO Rapid Assessment and Cause Finding Mission, 2 Novembere23 November 2007. World Health Organization, Geneva. Available at: https://www.who.int/csr/don/2007_11_16/en/.
- Guzewich, J.J., Bryan, F.L., Todd, E.C., 1997. Surveillance of foodborne disease I. Purposes and types of surveillance systems and networks. J. Food Protec. 60 (5), 555-556.
- WHO, 2008. Foodborne Disease Outbreaks e Guideline for Investigation and Control. Available at: https://www.who. int/foodsafety/publications/foodborne_disease/outbreak_guidelines.pdf.
- WHO, 2021. Manual for Investigating Suspected Outbreaks of Illnesses of Possible Chemical Etiology - Guidance for Investigation and Control. Available at: https://www.who.int/ipcs/ publications/en/.

Note: Ataxia is a lack of muscle coordination that may affect a person's speech, eye movements, and ability to swallow, walk, and pick up objects, among other voluntary movements.

9.10 Dilemma of cheese in a sack

In my professional career I have been faced with paradoxical situations, where on the one hand we are committed to preserving our cultural foods, but on the other hand we develop hygiene rules and legislation that run counter to these or are not feasible in the current socioeconomic context. An example of such a situation is cheese in a sack, a typical Herzegovinian product.

Cheese in a sack is a product made in the Dinaric mountain range for centuries. In Herzegovina, presence of this cheese dates back to the year 1379 (Samardzic et al., 2021). This product is unique and very different from all known cheeses due to one phase of its preparation, the ripening (60 days) takes place in smoked tanned sheepskin. This method probably was invented spontaneously with the purpose of conserving product for a longer period of time.

The cheese is made from raw cow's, sheep's, or goat's milk, or a mixture of these. The phases of cheese-making are curdling, draining, salting, pressing, breaking the cheese block into smaller pieces, inserting them into the sheepskin, and ripening. In the process of making cheese in a sack, nonstandard (unusual) means of work are used, such as sheepskin bag, cotton cloth for wrapping, a large stone for pressing, and a wooden plank. Moreover, the preparation of sheepskin is a cultural trade secret, a local know-how, passed from generation to generation. It cannot be replaced by a modern standard operation in a regular cheese-making process.

While at all levels of government, local and state, authorities declare to be committed to preserving local products, at the same time, the regulatory situation of products made of non-pasteurized milk is ambiguous, neither allowed nor prohibited legally. Also, changes in the production technology of traditional products would result in the loss of their uniqueness. Cheese in a sack cannot be made without the use of the sheepskin sack, which is a nonstandard material in cheese-making, nor from pasteurized milk because in that case it would lose microorganisms that give it a characteristic taste and smell during the ripening process. Also, small-scale family dairies will have difficulty fulfilling strict hygiene standards.

Discussion and key learnings

The case described here is an example of a dilemma. On the one hand, all efforts are made to preserve a unique local delicacy, while on the other hand legal requirements must be met and food safety assured. One of the main hazards in raw milk dairy products is brucellosis, but that has been found to be effectively eliminated after 60 days of ripening. Other countries have similar experiences with other products such as raw minced meat, i.e., steak tartare, raw eggs, or - in a somewhat similar situation - raw milk soft cheese (France).
Accepting that brucellosis can indeed be controlled through ripening (existing research may need to be reconfirmed in this particular environment), additional concerns, e.g., Listeria, will need to be controlled in other ways. That will involve food safety education at farm level dairies, rigorous microbiological monitoring, and upgrading of hygienic production conditions, including careful management of the health status of farm animals. In addition, legislation may have to be adapted to allow for carefully controlled production of this specialty cheese.

It will also require an initiative to raise consumer awareness on how such an age- old traditional product can be safely brought into the 21st century, retaining the key elements of the tradition, but now under carefully controlled conditions. For cheese in a sack, it will not be an easy journey, but Herzegovinians may still decide that their heritage is worth it.

References

Samardzic, S., Duric, G., Rudic-Grujic, V., Radovanovic, G., Dizdarevic, T., Dordevic- Milosevic, S., 2021. In: Gostin, A., Bogueva, D., Kakurinov, V. (Eds.), Nutritional and Health Aspects of the Food of the Balkans. Elsevier. https://www. elsevier.com/books/nutritional-and-health-aspects-of-food-in-the-balkans/gostin/978-0-12-820782-6.

Further reading

Gilman, H.L., Dahlberg, J, C., Marquardt, C., 1946. The occurrence and survival of Brucella abortus in cheddar and limburger cheese. J. of Dairy Sci. 29 (2), pp. 71-85. https:// www.sciencedirect.com/science/article/pii/S0022030246924484.

9.11 Safe first food innovating to tackle human milk scarcity

Thanks to creative use of social media, in 2010, two Canadian women led a global drive to ensure that caregivers of babies in need of human milk connect with mothers who are able to donate milk. Within 6 months, a vast commerce-free milk-sharing network was in place in some 50 countries and on every continent (Milk sharing, 2011).

However, this contemporary variation on a practice that is as old as our species instantly became the target of stern "Don't do it!" warnings from public health authorities. In addition, a number of influential associations representing pediatricians spoke out against informal human milk sharing as unsafe, insisting that mothers restrict their search to human milk banks. This attitude ignored a larger supply- and-demand reality. Simply put, there is not enough banked milk to meet the needs of even the sickest and most fragile babies.

Many mothers nevertheless continue their determined dissent from the artificial and unphysiological by securing and providing human milk, based on informed choice, for healthy babies who would otherwise be deprived.

Informed sharing of human milk, mother to mother, is an eloquent and compelling demonstration of who is in charge here. Although I had not given the topic much thought, I was among the early nonconformist observers who disagreed with the two interrelated fallacies being forcefully advanced by milk sharing critics:

- First, that mother-to-mother milk sharing is fundamentally riskier than feeding infant formula.

- Scond, that it is unfeasible for mothers, acting on their own, to minimize inherent health risks.

In addition, some observers expressed gloomy misgivings about the negative impact that informal milk sharing would have on human milk banking by worsening the already dire shortage of banked milk for the sickest and most fragile babies. Moreover, it was not unusual for the popular media to insinuate that informal sharing was equivalent to casual sharing.

I vigorously rejected this offensive and unfair characterization, which implies that mothers are not only acting recklessly but that they are also incapable of making informed choices. Make no mistake, I argued; no act could be more deliberate than mothers seeking a safe alternative natural supply of their babies' sole source of nourishment.

Since 2011, I have spoken and written on informed human milk sharing, including during in-person and online conferences attended mainly by health professionals and members of mother support groups. My focus was the convergence of knowledgeable and highly motivated women, reclaiming lost nurturing and nutritional ground by extending control over the availability and use of their milk and sharing it in a safe, ethical manner in the belief that they are capable of:

- Making informed choices, free of coercion
- Evaluating information on the benefits and risks
- Reducing exposure to pathogens, including by pasteurization

I sought to strike a balance between risks and benefits, reasoning that, since public health authorities routinely promote risk-reduction and harm-minimization strategies, it should be no different on behalf of babies lacking their own mothers' milk.

As to whether informal sharing threatened supply for donor milk banks, I observed that, in fact, each approach involved different groups of mothers and babies. Babies receiving banked donor milk were exclusively the sick and the hospitalized. In contrast, the milk being accessed mother to mother was for babies who did not usually qualify for banked donor milk.

Thus, direct mother-to-mother milk sharing should be viewed as complementary to donor milk banking and not as its competitor. Health authorities should examine the initiative closely, determine what is happening, and provide resources to make mother-to-mother milk sharing as safe as possible.
Finally, in 2018, an influential global organization of medical doctors - the Academy of Breastfeeding Medicine (ABM) - took a bold step to ensure that babies are safe, mothers are confident, and health professionals are enabled. Since its founding in 1993, the Academy has provided evidence-based solutions to challenges facing breastfeeding in support of its members in nearly 60 countries who are dedicated to protecting, promoting, and supporting breastfeeding.

In response to increased informal sharing of human milk, in January 2018, the Academy's authoritative peer-reviewed multidisciplinary journal, Breastfeeding Medicine, published detailed guidance for healthcare providers (Position Statement, 2017), so they can educate and support their patients about informal milk sharing. To summarize:

- The Academy's position statement focuses on two key strategies for maximizing the safety of community-based breast milk sharing: medical screening of the donor and safe milk-handling practices.

- Donors should have no medical illness where breastfeeding is contraindicated, nor should they be using any medication or herbal preparations which are incompatible with breastfeeding.
- Verification usually requires the review of a donor's medical history, including, where possible, her prenatal infectious screening tests and social practices.
- Healthcare providers can advise mothers who want to further reduce the risk of infections by performing home pasteurization. However, they should also be informed that pasteurization can significantly decrease the benefit of some human milk components.
- Responsibility for milk exchange remains with donors and recipients. Healthcare providers should instruct both donors and recipients on safe milk handling and storage practices.
- Internet-based breast milk sharing, and especially the purchase of milk over the Internet, is strongly discouraged since
- Donors are unknown to recipients and cannot be medically screened.
- The milk, upon arrival, is often unsuitable for consumption.

Two themes are conspicuously absent from the ABM position statement:

- There is no attempt to scold donor and recipient mothers, who are engaging in informed milk sharing, for somehow acting inappropriately.
- There is no accusation that informal milk sharing reduces the supply of milk from human milk banks for sick and hospitalized infants.

Discussion and key learnings

The global consensus could not be clearer (Global strategy, 2003). Breastfeeding is an unequaled way of providing ideal food for the healthy growth and development of infants, who should be exclusively breastfed for the first 6 months of life to achieve optimal growth, development, and health. Thereafter, to meet their evolving nutritional requirements, infants should receive nutritionally adequate and safe complementary foods while breastfeeding continues.

For those situations where infants are not breastfed, the choice of the best alternative - expressed breast milk from an infant's own mother, breast milk from a healthy wet nurse or a human milk bank, or a suitable breast milk substituted depends on individual circumstances.

In the context, the public health community has a choice: stay on the sidelines or move to engage by assisting those involved in milk sharing to make it as safe as possible. Engagement is called for in the belief that:

- Milk sharing will happen regardless of denunciations
- Its level of risk is manageable
- There are greater risks for babies who do not receive human milk

The made-by-mothers model described here shows great potential for expanding the world's supply of human milk and improving the health of children.

As to the first fallacy mentioned earlier - that mother-to-mother milk sharing is fundamentally riskier than feeding infant formula - it is important to recall the mass of scientific and epidemiological evidence not of the so-called benefits of breastfeeding but of the risks associated with being deprived of human milk.

Concerning the second fallacy - that it is unfeasible for mothers to satisfactorily minimize health risks - it is important to consider the following factors:

- Mothers who are donating milk are, or very recently have been, breastfeeding their own children.
- With few exceptions, these mothers are followed closely by healthcare professionals, with all that this implies in terms of health status monitoring.
- Generally, donor mothers are prepared to discuss their lifestyle and to share their medical records, one on one, before providing their milk to other mothers.

The milk sharing community provides mothers detailed risk-reduction guidance about informed choice, donor screening, safe milk handling, home pasteurization, and full disclosure. Today, I continue to emphatically affirm that:

- The two systems in place - protocol-driven human milk banks and unstructured informed mother-to-mother milk sharing - operate on parallel non-competitive tracks; they remain complementary, not antagonistic.
- There is significant untapped potential for both systems to play mutually supportive roles based on a common objective: that no babies are denied their nurturing and nutritional birthright.

Tension between health authorities, milk banks, and milk sharing networks is inevitable only if the parties remain isolated and fail to communicate. With this common objective in mind, dialogue and collaboration can sensibly lead to development of realistic guidelines enabling health professionals, whether acting in a hospital setting or in the community, to advise and support the families in their care.

The position statement of the ABM on informal breast milk sharing for the term healthy infant is at once clear, concise, and unequivocal. It is up to public health authorities, including associations of healthcare providers, to give it practical effect on behalf of those mothers and babies in need.

References

Global Strategy for Infant and Young Child Feeding, 2003. World Health Organization. https://www.who.int/publications/i/item/9241562218.

Further reading

- Akre, J., Gribble, K.D., Minchin, M., 2011. Milk sharing: from private practice to public pursuit. Int. Breastfeed. J. 6, 8 (2011). http://www.internationalbreastfeedingjournal.com/content/6/1/8.
- Sriraman, Natasha K. et al, Academy of Breastfeeding Medicine's 2017 Position Statement on Informal Breast Milk Sharing for the Term Healthy Infant,
- Breastfeeding Medicine 2018 13:1, 2-4, https://www.liebertpub.com/doi/10.1089/bfm.2017.29064.nks.

Epilogue

Dear readers,

In the day-to-day practice of food safety, things can go wrong. We may learn about it in the news, when products are recalled, people and companies are prosecuted, but we don't always get the inside story. All over the world, food safety training is provided, but the use of inside accounts of actual cases is rare. This book has collected a number of those stories, the real-life mishaps and mistakes in the public health sector or food industry, for the benefit of the training and education of food professionals and those interested in the field of food safety.

The stories cover the whole range of measures from basic hygiene practice, such as handwashing or hygienic design of equipment, to the final safety valve of food safety management systems: whistleblowing – and everything in between. They:

- Illustrate the challenges that food and public health professionals are facing in raising awareness of the importance of food safety and promoting collaboration across disciplines, reminding us of the interdisciplinary nature of the subject.
- Highlight the importance of management commitment, corporate culture and professional ethics, including the dilemmas we may sometimes face in the decision-making process.
- Illustrate the various risks, how people have successfully addressed them through food hygiene measures and proficient management or failed to do so.
- Report accounts of incidents, their investigation and their learnings.
- Address issues of communication between professionals or with consumers. We show that understanding perceptions

is essential to managing food safety. There is often a huge disconnect between people's perceptions and the hard facts of food safety, both in terms of what is perceived as safe but is not. And vice versa, what is considered dangerous but would not have a significant public health impact.

The take-home message of this book is that food safety management, like most things in life, is a human activity. Science, methods, laws and standards are central to food safety, but they may only be effective in a conducive environment. Working conditions and employees'/managers' attitude and ethics play a central role in assuring the safety of products. As a number of stories illustrate, where people work under duress, e.g., lack of time, shortage of tools/resources, expertise, experience, interest/motivation, or when they have to follow unfeasible instructions, mistakes will be made for which consumers and employers will bear the consequences. These examples support the current international emphasis on "food safety culture" including proper regulations and protections around whistleblowing.

On this occasion, we would like to thank all the contributors for having shared their professional experiences and collaborated in preparing this book.

We look forward to receiving feedback from readers.

Acknowledgements

The authors wish to thank the following people for their valuable contributions:

James Akre, BA, MPIA, freelance author, speaker, reviewer and commentator on the sociocultural dimension of breastfeeding, Geneva, Switzerland

Abenaa Akyaa Okyere (Mrs), Ghana Atomic Energy Commission, Biotechnology & Nuclear Agriculture Research Institute, Ghana

Asst. Prof. Dr. Murat Ay, Doğuş University, Gastronomy and Culinary Arts Department, İstanbul, Turkey

Prof. Dr. Diána Bánáti , Full Professor, Vice Dean, Faculty of Engineering, University of Szeged, Hungary

Vương Bảo Thy, Ph.D., Head of Faculty of Health Sciences, University of Cuu Long, 1A Highway, Phu Quoi, Long Ho, Vinh Long 8500, Viet Nam

Sarah Blanchard, Food Safety Specialist

Daniela Borda, Professor, Faculty of Food Science and Engineering, "Dunărea de Jos" University of Galaţi, Romania

John Carter: VP Quality and Food Safety, former board member of GFSI.

Suchart Chaven, PepsiCo Beverage Food Safety Director

D. D. O. Cromie

Juliane Dias, Quality and Food Safety Comunicator Flavor Food Consulting

D. J. Dearden

Bas van Driel, MBA, laboratory expert

Dr. Ir. Gerrit van Duijn, Vlaardingen, The Netherlands

Julio Egocheaga, Dr. Eng.

Dr. Matilda Freund, Vice President, Global Food Safety, Mondelēz International, Switzerland

Asst. Prof. Dr. İsmail Hakkı Tekiner, İstanbul Sabahattin Zaim University, Food and Nutrition Department, İstanbul, Turkey

Lynne B. Hare, Ph.D., Fellow, American Statistical Association, Fellow, American Society for Quality, Statistical Engineer, Statistical Strategies, LLC

Prof. John Holah, Principal Corporate Scientist, Kersia Group

Saint Yi Htet, Food Safety Specialist

Aline Issa, Ph.D., Holy Spirit University of Kaslik (USEK), Lebanon

Dr.med.vet. Fritz K. Käferstein, Director and Professor, former Director of Programme of Food Safety and Food Aid, World Health Organization, Geneva, Switzerland

Prof. Dr Vladimir Kakurinov, GHI Ambassador for Macedonia

Antonio Khabbaz, Agri-food Engineer/University Lecturer (USEK, AUB, ULS), Lead auditor – Food Safety Management Systems (FSMS), Lead trainer – Food Safety Preventive Control Alliance (FDA – FSMA)

Sagar Mahmood Khan, Food Safety Expert, Pakistan

Ron Milewski, Kraft Foods

Gerald G. Moy, Ph.D., Formerly GEMS/Food Manager Department of Food Safety and Zoonoses World Health Organization, Geneva, Switzerland

David Napper

Anca Ioana Nicolau, Professor, Faculty of Food Science and Engineering, "Dunărea de Jos" University of Galaţi, Romania

Assist. prof. Andrej Ovca, PhD, University of Ljubljana, Faculty of Health Sciences, Ljubljana, Slovenia

K. T. Rowlands

Dr Slavica Samardzic, Ministry of agriculture, forestry and water management of Republic of Srpska, Banja Luka, Republic of Srpska, Bosnia and Herzegovina, and Slow Food Convivium Trebinje, Republic of Srpska, Bosnia and Herzegovina

Dr. Rudolf Schmitt, University of Applied Science of Western Switzerland, Sion, Switzerland

F. Tracy Schonrock, Retired from the U. S. Department of Agriculture, Agricultural Marketing Service, Dairy Inspection and Grading Branch, Affiliations: EHEDG, 3-A SSI, NSF International, Alpha Zeta Honorary Fraternity, Fairfax Station, VA USA

Dr Alexandrina Sirbu, Professor "Constantin Brancoveanu" University of Pitesti (UCB), FMMAE Ramnicu Valcea, Valcea County, Romania

Joe Stout RS – Founder Commercial Food Sanitation

Dr John Yew Huat Tang, Associate Professor Faculty of Bioresources and Food Industry, Universiti

Sultan Zainal Abidin (Besut Campus), 22200 Besut, Terengganu, Malaysia

Paula Teixeira, Universidade Católica Portuguesa, CBQF - Centro de Biotecnologia e Química Fina – Laboratório Associado, Escola Superior de Biotecnologia, Rua Diogo Botelho 1327, 4169-005 Porto, Portugal

Lara Hanna-Wakim, Professor of Food Process Engineering, Department of Agricultural and Food Sciences, Holy Spirit University of Kaslik (USEK), Lebanon

Chin-Kun Wang, Former President & Distinguished Professor, Chung Shan Medical University, Taiwan

Marc Bou Zeidan, Associate Professor of Microbiology and Biotechnology, Department of Agricultural and Food Sciences, Holy Spirit University of Kaslik (USEK), Lebanon

Index

www.ingramcontent.com/pod-product-compliance
Lightning Source LLC
Chambersburg PA
CBHW021436180326
41458CB00001B/300